NURSING ASSISTANT
SKILLS CHECKLIST

NURSING ASSISTANT
SKILLS CHECKLIST

Trisha Kennamer
Mike Kennamer

THOMSON

DELMAR LEARNING

Australia   Canada   Mexico   Singapore   Spain   United Kingdom   United States

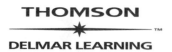

THOMSON

DELMAR LEARNING

Nursing Assistant Skills Checklist
Prepared by Trisha Kennamer and Mike Kennamer

Vice President, Health Care Business Unit:
William Brottmiller

Editorial Director:
Cathy L. Esperti

Acquisitions Editor:
Marah Bellegarde

Developmental Editor:
Sherry Conners

Editorial Assistant:
Jadin Babin-Kavanaugh

Marketing Director:
Jennifer McAvey

Marketing Coordinator:
Michele Gleason

Production Editor:
Anne Sherman

Library of Congress Cataloging-in-Publication Data

Kennamer, Trisha.
 Nursing assistant skills checklist / prepared by Trisha Kennamer, Mike Kennamer.
  p. ; cm.
 Includes bibliographical references and index.
  ISBN 1-4018-7193-3 (alk. paper)
 1. Nurses' aides—Handbooks, manuals, etc. 2. Nursing—Handbooks, manuals, etc.
 [DNLM: 1. Nurses' Aides—Handbooks. 2. Nursing Care—methods—Handbooks. 3. Clinical Competence—Handbooks.]
 I. Kennamer, Mike. II. Title.

 RT84.K466 2006
 610.73'06'98—dc22

                    2005004034

Notice to the Reader

CONTENTS

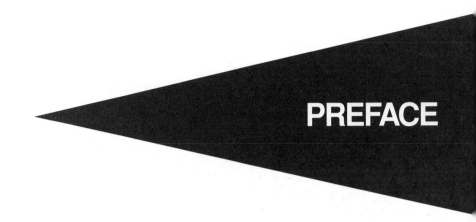

Nursing Assistant Skills Checklist is a compilation of checklists detailing the steps required to perform over 160 procedures. This product can be used as a tool for those who are studying to be nursing assistants; by instructors who want a tool to check student competency; or within an in-service training environment at the workplace.

Features and Benefits:

- Procedure checklists include the beginning and ending procedure so crucial in the health care environment.
- Checklists include a section for instructor or student comments.
- Three-hole punched and perforated so the pages can easily be removed as required by the instructor.
- Can be used as an accompaniment to any nursing assistant product.

Also Available:

Competency Exam Prep and Review for Nursing Assistants
0766814297

This comprehensive self-study book reviews all the basic skills that a nursing assistant must know to pass the certification examination.

Nurse Aide Exam Review Cards
1401808336

Nurse Aide Exam Review Cards with Audio CD-Rom
140180831X

Nurse Aide Exam Review Cards, Spanish Edition
1401808328

This covers all the basic skills a nursing assistant needs to pass the certification exam. Each page contains four cards that can be easily separated to become flash cards.

On the Job: The Essentials of Nursing Assisting
1401806457

Here is a pocket-sized reference guide for the nursing assistant to use once hired. This guide includes important information such as A Patient Bill of Rights and difficult or special procedures that the nursing assistant may perform on the job.

Acknowledgments:

Thomson Delmar Learning and the authors wish to thank the following reviewers for their input in the development of this book:

Susan Lewsen, MA, BSN, RN
Davis Applied Technology College
Kaysville, UT

Cindy Scott, RN, BSN
Kirkwood Community College
Cedar Rapids, IA

Ann Sims, RN
Albuquerque Technical Vocational Institute
Albuquerque, NM

Checklist for Beginning Procedure Actions

Name _____ Date _____

School _____

Instructor _____

Course _____

Beginning Procedure Actions	Able to Perform	Able to Perform with Assistance	Unable to Perform	Initials and Date
1. Wash your hands. *Comments:*	☐	☐	☐	
2. Provide privacy. *Comments:*	☐	☐	☐	
3. Explain what will happen and answer any questions. *Comments:*	☐	☐	☐	
4. Allow the patient to assist as much as possible. *Comments:*	☐	☐	☐	
5. Raise the bed to a comfortable working height. *Comments:*	☐	☐	☐	
6. Lower the side rail on the side you will be working. *Comments:*	☐	☐	☐	
7. Position the patient for the procedure. *Comments:*	☐	☐	☐	
8. Drape the patient for modesty. *Comments:*	☐	☐	☐	
9. Set up equipment at the bedside. *Comments:*	☐	☐	☐	
10. Carry out precaution gowning and gloving. *Comments:*	☐	☐	☐	

Checklist for Procedure Completion Actions

Name _____ Date _____

School _____

Instructor _____

Course _____

Procedure Completion Actions	Able to Perform	Able to Perform with Assistance	Unable to Perform	Initials and Date
1. Remove gloves. *Comments:*	☐	☐	☐	
2. Position the patient comfortably. *Comments:*	☐	☐	☐	
3. Replace the bed covers. *Comments:*	☐	☐	☐	
4. Remove any drapes, if used. *Comments:*	☐	☐	☐	
5. Return the bed to the lowest horizontal position. *Comments:*	☐	☐	☐	
6. Elevate the side rails. *Comments:*	☐	☐	☐	
7. Leave the signal cord within easy reach of the patient. *Comments:*	☐	☐	☐	
8. Perform a general safety check. *Comments:*	☐	☐	☐	
9. Open the privacy curtains. *Comments:*	☐	☐	☐	
10. Remove and discard personal protective equipment (PPE). *Comments:*	☐	☐	☐	
11. Care for equipment according to policy. *Comments:*	☐	☐	☐	

continued on the following page

continued from the previous page

Procedure Completion Actions	Able to Perform	Able to Perform with Assistance	Unable to Perform	Initials and Date
12. Wash your hands. *Comments:*	☐	☐	☐	
13. Let visitors know they may reenter the room. *Comments:*	☐	☐	☐	
14. Report completion of task. *Comments:*	☐	☐	☐	
15. Document actions and your observation. *Comments:*	☐	☐	☐	

Checklist for Procedure 1   Handwashing

Name _____ Date _____

School _____

Instructor _____

Course _____

Procedure 1 Handwashing	Able to Perform	Able to Perform with Assistance	Unable to Perform	Initials and Date
1. Check to ensure there is adequate soap and towel supply. *Comments:*	☐	☐	☐	
2. Remove your rings and watch. *Comments:*	☐	☐	☐	
3. Turn on the faucet with a dry paper towel and discard the towel in a waste container. *Comments:*	☐	☐	☐	
4. Adjust water to a warm temperature. *Comments:*	☐	☐	☐	
5. Apply soap and lather. *Comments:*	☐	☐	☐	
6. Rinse hands. *Comments:*	☐	☐	☐	
7. Dry hands and discard towel into a waste container. *Comments:*	☐	☐	☐	
8. Turn off faucet with a clean paper towel and discard into a waste container. *Comments:*	☐	☐	☐	
9. Apply lotion to hands. *Comments:*	☐	☐	☐	

Checklist for Procedure 2   Putting on a Mask

Name _____   Date _____

School _____

Instructor _____

Course _____

Procedure 2 **Putting on a Mask**	Able to Perform	Able to Perform with Assistance	Unable to Perform	Initials and Date
1. Assemble equipment. *Comments:*	☐	☐	☐	
2. Adjust the mask over your nose and mouth. *Comments:*	☐	☐	☐	
3. Tie the top strings first, then the bottom strings. *Comments:*	☐	☐	☐	

Checklist for Procedure 3   Putting on a Gown

Name _____ Date _____

School _____

Instructor _____

Course _____

Procedure 3 **Putting on a Gown**	Able to Perform	Able to Perform with Assistance	Unable to Perform	Initials and Date
1. Assemble equipment. *Comments:*	☐	☐	☐	
2. Remove your wristwatch and place on paper towel. *Comments:*	☐	☐	☐	
3. Wash hands. *Comments:*	☐	☐	☐	
4. Apply the mask first, if used. *Comments:*	☐	☐	☐	
5. Apply the gown. *Comments:*	☐	☐	☐	
6. Secure the neckband. *Comments:*	☐	☐	☐	
7. Secure the waist ties. *Comments:*	☐	☐	☐	

Checklist for Procedure 4   Putting on Gloves

Name _____   Date _____

School _____

Instructor _____

Course _____

Procedure 4 Putting on Gloves	Able to Perform	Able to Perform with Assistance	Unable to Perform	Initials and Date
1. Assemble equipment. *Comments:*	☐	☐	☐	
2. Wash hands. *Comments:*	☐	☐	☐	
3. Pick up the glove by the cuff and place on the other hand. *Comments:*	☐	☐	☐	
4. Repeat for the other hand. *Comments:*	☐	☐	☐	
5. Adjust gloves. *Comments:*	☐	☐	☐	

Checklist for Procedure 5   Removing Contaminated Gloves

Name _____ Date _____

School _____

Instructor _____

Course _____

Procedure 5 Removing Contaminated Gloves	Able to Perform	Able to Perform with Assistance	Unable to Perform	Initials and Date
1. Grasp the cuff of one glove on the outside with fingers of the other hand. *Comments:*	☐	☐	☐	
2. Pull the cuff of the glove down and remove. *Comments:*	☐	☐	☐	
3. Hold the glove with the still-gloved hand. *Comments:*	☐	☐	☐	
4. Insert finger of ungloved hand under the cuff of glove on the other hand. *Comments:*	☐	☐	☐	
5. Pull the glove off inside out. *Comments:*	☐	☐	☐	
6. Drop the gloves into biohazard waste receptacle. *Comments:*	☐	☐	☐	
7. Wash hands. *Comments:*	☐	☐	☐	

Checklist for Procedure 6   Removing Contaminated Gloves, Mask, and Gown

Name _____   Date _____

School _____

Instructor _____

Course _____

Procedure 6 **Removing Contaminated Gloves, Mask, and Gown**	Able to Perform	Able to Perform with Assistance	Unable to Perform	Initials and Date
1. Assemble equipment. *Comments:*	☐	☐	☐	
2. Remove gloves. *Comments:*	☐	☐	☐	
3. Undo waist ties of the gown. *Comments:*	☐	☐	☐	
4. Turn the faucets on with a clean paper towel and discard. *Comments:*	☐	☐	☐	
5. Wash and dry hands. *Comments:*	☐	☐	☐	
6. Turn off the faucets. *Comments:*	☐	☐	☐	
7. Remove and discard goggles, if used. *Comments:*	☐	☐	☐	
8. Remove the mask and dispose of it. *Comments:*	☐	☐	☐	
9. Undo the neckties and loosen the gown at shoulders. *Comments:*	☐	☐	☐	
10. Slip the fingers of your dominant hand inside the cuff of the other hand without touching the outside of the gown. *Comments:*	☐	☐	☐	

continued on the following page

continued from the previous page

Procedure 6	Able to Perform	Able to Perform with Assistance	Unable to Perform	Initials and Date
11. Using the gown-covered hand, pull the gown down over the dominant hand and then off of both arms. *Comments:*	☐	☐	☐	
12. Fold it away from the body, the contaminated side inward. Roll up the gown and dispose of it. *Comments:*	☐	☐	☐	
13. Wash hands. *Comments:*	☐	☐	☐	
14. If your watch was brought into area, remove it from the paper towel. Hold the clean side of the paper towel and dispose of it. *Comments:*	☐	☐	☐	
15. Use a paper towel to grasp the door handle as you leave. Dispose of the paper towel before you leave the room. *Comments:*	☐	☐	☐	

Checklist for Procedure 7 Serving a Meal in an Isolation Unit

Name _____ Date _____

School _____

Instructor _____

Course _____

Procedure 7 Serving a Meal in an Isolation Unit	Able to Perform	Able to Perform with Assistance	Unable to Perform	Initials and Date
1. Wash hands. Comments:	☐	☐	☐	
2. Obtain meal tray. Comments:	☐	☐	☐	
3. Ask for assistance. Comments:	☐	☐	☐	
4. Place the tray on the isolation cart. Comments:	☐	☐	☐	
5. Put on personal protective equipment (PPE). Comments:	☐	☐	☐	
6. Enter the room and identify the patient. Comments:	☐	☐	☐	
7. Explain what you plan to do. Comments:	☐	☐	☐	
8. Provide privacy. Comments:	☐	☐	☐	
9. Raise the bed. Comments:	☐	☐	☐	
10. Pick up the meal tray that remains in the room. Comments:	☐	☐	☐	
11. Go to the door and open it with a paper towel. Comments:	☐	☐	☐	
12. Carefully transfer items to the isolation tray. Comments:	☐	☐	☐	

continued on the following page

continued from the previous page

Procedure 7	Able to Perform	Able to Perform with Assistance	Unable to Perform	Initials and Date
13. Place the isolation tray on the overbed table. *Comments:*	☐	☐	☐	
14. Prepare the patient for the meal. *Comments:*	☐	☐	☐	
15. Check the patient's identification band against the meal tray card. *Comments:*	☐	☐	☐	
16. Assist the patient as needed. *Comments:*	☐	☐	☐	
17. Note how much food and liquid have been eaten. *Comments:*	☐	☐	☐	
18. Place all disposable items in appropriate waste receptacle. *Comments:*	☐	☐	☐	
19. Use a paper towel to open the door. *Comments:*	☐	☐	☐	
20. Prop the door open with your foot. *Comments:*	☐	☐	☐	
21. Transfer reusable dishes to the tray held by an assistant. *Comments:*	☐	☐	☐	
22. Clean the isolation meal tray and store in the isolation unit. *Comments:*	☐	☐	☐	
23. Carry out procedure completion actions. *Comments:*	☐	☐	☐	
24. Remove PPE and discard. *Comments:*	☐	☐	☐	
25. Wash hands. *Comments:*	☐	☐	☐	
26. Open the door with a paper towel and discard it before leaving the unit. *Comments:*	☐	☐	☐	

Checklist for Procedure 8   Measuring Vital Signs in an Isolation Unit

Name _____ Date _____

School _____

Instructor _____

Course _____

Procedure 8 **Measuring Vital Signs in an Isolation Unit**	Able to Perform	Able to Perform with Assistance	Unable to Perform	Initials and Date
1. Wash hands. *Comments:*	☐	☐	☐	
2. Remove your wristwatch and place on a clean paper towel. *Comments:*	☐	☐	☐	
3. Put on personal protective equipment (PPE). *Comments:*	☐	☐	☐	
4. Pick up the paper towel that contains the watch. *Comments:*	☐	☐	☐	
5. Enter the isolation unit. Open the door with a paper towel. *Comments:*	☐	☐	☐	
6. Place the watch where it can be seen. *Comments:*	☐	☐	☐	
7. Identify the patient and explain what you are about to do. *Comments:*	☐	☐	☐	
8. Provide privacy. *Comments:*	☐	☐	☐	
9. Allow the patient to help as much as possible. *Comments:*	☐	☐	☐	
10. Raise the bed. *Comments:*	☐	☐	☐	
11. Measure vital signs, using the patient's dedicated equipment. *Comments:*	☐	☐	☐	

continued on the following page

continued from the previous page

Procedure 8	Able to Perform	Able to Perform with Assistance	Unable to Perform	Initials and Date
12. Note the readings. *Comments:*	☐	☐	☐	
13. Clean and store equipment. *Comments:*	☐	☐	☐	
14. Carry out all procedure completion actions. *Comments:*	☐	☐	☐	
15. Wash hands; dry them and pick up your watch. *Comments:*	☐	☐	☐	
16. Discard the paper towel. *Comments:*	☐	☐	☐	
17. Pick up the notes. *Comments:*	☐	☐	☐	
18. Open the door with a paper towel and discard it before leaving the unit. *Comments:*	☐	☐	☐	

Checklist for Procedure 9   Transferring Nondisposable Equipment Outside of Isolation Unit

Name _____ Date _____

School _____

Instructor _____

Course _____

Procedure 9 **Transferring Nondisposable Equipment** **Outside of Isolation Unit**	Able to Perform	Able to Perform with Assistance	Unable to Perform	Initials and Date
1. Clean equipment with disinfectant before leaving the unit. *Comments:*	☐	☐	☐	
2. Place equipment in biohazard plastic bag. *Comments:*	☐	☐	☐	
3. Remove the contaminated gloves, mask, and gown. *Comments:*	☐	☐	☐	
4. Pick up the bag containing equipment and leave isolation unit. *Comments:*	☐	☐	☐	

Checklist for Procedure 10   Specimen Collection from a Patient in an Isolation Unit

Name _____ Date _____

School _____

Instructor _____

Course _____

Procedure 10 **Specimen Collection from a Patient in an Isolation Unit**	Able to Perform	Able to Perform with Assistance	Unable to Perform	Initials and Date
1. Assemble equipment. *Comments:*	☐	☐	☐	
2. Put on personal protective equipment (PPE). *Comments:*	☐	☐	☐	
3. Keep the biohazard bag for specimen transport outside isolation unit. *Comments:*	☐	☐	☐	
4. Carry equipment into isolation unit. *Comments:*	☐	☐	☐	
5. Place the container and cover on a paper towel. *Comments:*	☐	☐	☐	
6. Identify the patient and explain what you plan to do. *Comments:*	☐	☐	☐	
7. Provide privacy. *Comments:*	☐	☐	☐	
8. Allow the patient to help as much as possible. *Comments:*	☐	☐	☐	
9. Raise the bed. *Comments:*	☐	☐	☐	
10. Place the specimen into the container without touching the outside. *Comments:*	☐	☐	☐	

continued on the following page

continued from the previous page

Procedure 10	Able to Perform	Able to Perform with Assistance	Unable to Perform	Initials and Date
11. Cover the container and apply a label. *Comments:*	☐	☐	☐	
12. Clean equipment. *Comments:*	☐	☐	☐	
13. Remove PPE. *Comments:*	☐	☐	☐	
14. Wash hands. *Comments:*	☐	☐	☐	
15. Use a paper towel to pick up the specimen container. *Comments:*	☐	☐	☐	
16. Open the door with a clean paper towel. Outside the unit gather the towel inside your hand so the edges do not hang loosely. *Comments:*	☐	☐	☐	
17. Place the specimen container in biohazard transport bag. *Comments:*	☐	☐	☐	
18. Discard the paper towels. *Comments:*	☐	☐	☐	
19. Transport the specimen. *Comments:*	☐	☐	☐	
20. Wash hands. *Comments:*	☐	☐	☐	

Checklist for Procedure 11   Caring for Linens in an Isolation Unit

Name _____ Date _____

School _____

Instructor _____

Course _____

Procedure 11 Caring for Linens in an Isolation Unit	Able to Perform	Able to Perform with Assistance	Unable to Perform	Initials and Date
1. Assemble linen and place on a chair or a stand outside the isolation unit. *Comments:*	☐	☐	☐	
2. Wash and dry hands. *Comments:*	☐	☐	☐	
3. Put on personal protective equipment (PPE). *Comments:*	☐	☐	☐	
4. Open the door with a paper towel. *Comments:*	☐	☐	☐	
5. Once inside the isolation unit, place the clean linen on a chair. *Comments:*	☐	☐	☐	
6. Identify the patient and explain what you plan to do. *Comments:*	☐	☐	☐	
7. Provide privacy. *Comments:*	☐	☐	☐	
8. Allow the patient to help as much as possible. *Comments:*	☐	☐	☐	
9. Raise the bed. *Comments:*	☐	☐	☐	
10. Remove the soiled linen from the bed. *Comments:*	☐	☐	☐	

continued on the following page

continued from the previous page

Procedure 11	Able to Perform	Able to Perform with Assistance	Unable to Perform	Initials and Date
11. Place the soiled linen in a melt-away laundry bag or follow facility policy. *Comments:*	☐	☐	☐	
12. Label the bag as biohazard material. *Comments:*	☐	☐	☐	
13. Place the bag in the hamper. *Comments:*	☐	☐	☐	
14. Secure the bag and route to laundry. *Comments:*	☐	☐	☐	
15. Remove gloves if soiled. *Comments:*	☐	☐	☐	
16. Wash hands; put on clean gloves. *Comments:*	☐	☐	☐	
17. Remake the bed. *Comments:*	☐	☐	☐	
18. Carry out all procedure completion actions. *Comments:*	☐	☐	☐	

Checklist for Procedure 12 Transporting Patient to and from Isolation Unit

Name _____ Date _____

School _____

Instructor _____

Course _____

Procedure 12 **Transporting Patient to and from Isolation Unit**	Able to Perform	Able to Perform with Assistance	Unable to Perform	Initials and Date
1. Wash hands. *Comments:*	☐	☐	☐	
2. Assemble equipment. *Comments:*	☐	☐	☐	
3. Notify the department that a patient from isolation unit is being transported to them. *Comments:*	☐	☐	☐	
4. Ask for assistance, if needed. *Comments:*	☐	☐	☐	
5. Cover the transport vehicle with a clean sheet. *Comments:*	☐	☐	☐	
6. Wash hands. *Comments:*	☐	☐	☐	
7. Put on PPE. *Comments:*	☐	☐	☐	
8. Wheel the transport vehicle into the isolation unit. *Comments:*	☐	☐	☐	
9. Opening the door with a paper towel. *Comments:*	☐	☐	☐	
10. Identify the patient and explain what you plan to do. *Comments:*	☐	☐	☐	

continued on the following page

continued from the previous page

Procedure 12	Able to Perform	Able to Perform with Assistance	Unable to Perform	Initials and Date
11. Provide privacy. *Comments:*	☐	☐	☐	
12. Allow the patient to help as much as possible. *Comments:*	☐	☐	☐	
13. Raise or lower the bed depending upon the transport vehicle. *Comments:*	☐	☐	☐	
14. Assist the patient to transport vehicle. *Comments:*	☐	☐	☐	
15. Put a mask on the patient, if required. *Comments:*	☐	☐	☐	
16. Wrap the patient in a sheet, if required. *Comments:*	☐	☐	☐	
17. Remove PPE. *Comments:*	☐	☐	☐	
18. Wash hands. *Comments:*	☐	☐	☐	
19. Open the door with a paper towel and transport the patient out of the isolation unit. *Comments:*	☐	☐	☐	
20. To return a patient to the isolation unit, put on PPE. *Comments:*	☐	☐	☐	
21. Enter the isolation unit. *Comments:*	☐	☐	☐	
22. Unwrap the patient and remove his mask. *Comments:*	☐	☐	☐	
23. Assist the patient to return to bed. *Comments:*	☐	☐	☐	

Procedure 12	Able to Perform	Able to Perform with Assistance	Unable to Perform	Initials and Date
24. Carry out procedure completion actions. *Comments:*	☐	☐	☐	
25. Place the sheet in the laundry hamper. *Comments:*	☐	☐	☐	
26. Dispose of the patient's mask. *Comments:*	☐	☐	☐	
27. Remove PPE. *Comments:*	☐	☐	☐	
28. Wash hands. *Comments:*	☐	☐	☐	
29. Remove the transport vehicle by opening the door with a paper towel. *Comments:*	☐	☐	☐	
30. Report completion of procedure. *Comments:*	☐	☐	☐	

Checklist for Procedure 13   Opening a Sterile Package

Name _____ Date _____

School _____

Instructor _____

Course _____

Procedure 13 Opening a Sterile Package	Able to Perform	Able to Perform with Assistance	Unable to Perform	Initials and Date
1. Wash hands. Comments:	☐	☐	☐	
2. Assemble equipment. Comments:	☐	☐	☐	
3. Place the package with fold side up on a clean, flat surface. Comments:	☐	☐	☐	
4. Remove the tape. Comments:	☐	☐	☐	
5. Unfold the farthest away flap. Comments:	☐	☐	☐	
6. Open the right flap. Comments:	☐	☐	☐	
7. Open the left flap. Comments:	☐	☐	☐	
8. Open the final flap. Comments:	☐	☐	☐	

Checklist for Procedure 14   Turning the Patient toward You

Name _____ Date _____

School _____

Instructor _____

Course _____

Procedure 14 Turning the Patient toward You	Able to Perform	Able to Perform with Assistance	Unable to Perform	Initials and Date
1. Carry out beginning procedure actions. *Comments:*	☐	☐	☐	
2. Lower nearest side rail. *Comments:*	☐	☐	☐	
3. Cross far arm over the patient's chest. *Comments:*	☐	☐	☐	
4. Bend near arm at the elbow, bring hand toward the head of the bed. *Comments:*	☐	☐	☐	
5. Place your hand on the patient's far shoulder. *Comments:*	☐	☐	☐	
6. Place other hand on the patient's hips. *Comments:*	☐	☐	☐	
7. Brace thighs against the bed. *Comments:*	☐	☐	☐	
8. Roll the patient toward you. *Comments:*	☐	☐	☐	
9. Bring the patient's upper leg toward you and bend comfortably. *Comments:*	☐	☐	☐	
10. Put up the side rail. *Comments:*	☐	☐	☐	

continued on the following page

continued from the previous page

Procedure 14	Able to Perform	Able to Perform with Assistance	Unable to Perform	Initials and Date
11. Go to the opposite side of the bed. *Comments:*	☐	☐	☐	
12. Place hands under the patient's shoulders and then hips. *Comments:*	☐	☐	☐	
13. Pull toward the center of the bed. *Comments:*	☐	☐	☐	
14. Make sure the patient's body is properly aligned and safely positioned. *Comments:*	☐	☐	☐	
15. Place a pillow behind the patient's back if needed. *Comments:*	☐	☐	☐	
16. Position arms and legs if the patient is unable to do so. *Comments:*	☐	☐	☐	
17. Provide support with pillows to the shoulders, hands, knees, and ankles. *Comments:*	☐	☐	☐	
18. Carry out procedure completion actions. *Comments:*	☐	☐	☐	

Checklist for Procedure 15   Turning the Patient away from You

Name _____ Date _____

School _____

Instructor _____

Course _____

Procedure 15 Turning the Patient away from You	Able to Perform	Able to Perform with Assistance	Unable to Perform	Initials and Date
1. Carry out beginning procedure actions. *Comments:*	☐	☐	☐	
2. Lower the side rail. *Comments:*	☐	☐	☐	
3. Have the patient bend her knees. *Comments:*	☐	☐	☐	
4. Cross the patient's arms on her chest. *Comments:*	☐	☐	☐	
5. Place your arm under the patient's head and shoulder. *Comments:*	☐	☐	☐	
6. Place other hand and forearm under the small of the patient's back. *Comments:*	☐	☐	☐	
7. Bend your body at the hips and knees. *Comments:*	☐	☐	☐	
8. Pull the patient toward the edge of bed. *Comments:*	☐	☐	☐	
9. Place forearms under the patient's hips and pull toward you. *Comments:*	☐	☐	☐	
10. Move ankles and knees toward you. *Comments:*	☐	☐	☐	

continued on the following page

continued from the previous page

Procedure 15	Able to Perform	Able to Perform with Assistance	Unable to Perform	Initials and Date
11. Cross the near leg over the other leg. *Comments:*	☐	☐	☐	
12. Roll the patient away from you. *Comments:*	☐	☐	☐	
13. Place your hands under the patient's head and shoulders. *Comments:*	☐	☐	☐	
14. Draw the patient toward the center of the bed. *Comments:*	☐	☐	☐	
15. Move the patient's hips to the center of the bed. *Comments:*	☐	☐	☐	
16. Place a pillow behind the patient's back. *Comments:*	☐	☐	☐	
17. Check the patient's body position. *Comments:*	☐	☐	☐	
18. Replace the side rail. *Comments:*	☐	☐	☐	
19. Lower the bed to the lowest position. *Comments:*	☐	☐	☐	
20. Carry out procedure completion actions. *Comments:*	☐	☐	☐	

Checklist for Procedure 16   Moving a Patient to the Head of the Bed

Name _____ Date _____

School _____

Instructor _____

Course _____

Procedure 16 Moving a Patient to the Head of the Bed	Able to Perform	Able to Perform with Assistance	Unable to Perform	Initials and Date
1. Carry out beginning procedure actions. *Comments:*	☐	☐	☐	
2. Ask for assistance. *Comments:*	☐	☐	☐	
3. Lock the wheels of the bed. *Comments:*	☐	☐	☐	
4. Raise the bed to a comfortable working height. *Comments:*	☐	☐	☐	
5. Lower the side rails. *Comments:*	☐	☐	☐	
6. Lower the head of the bed and remove the pillow. *Comments:*	☐	☐	☐	
7. Lift the top bedding and expose the draw sheet. *Comments:*	☐	☐	☐	
8. Loosen the sides of the draw sheet. *Comments:*	☐	☐	☐	
9. Roll the draw sheet edges close to the patient's body. *Comments:*	☐	☐	☐	
10. Face the foot of bed. *Comments:*	☐	☐	☐	
11. Grasp the draw sheet. *Comments:*	☐	☐	☐	

continued on the following page

continued from the previous page

Procedure 16	Able to Perform	Able to Perform with Assistance	Unable to Perform	Initials and Date
12. Position feet 12 inches apart. *Comments:*	☐	☐	☐	
13. Place free hand and arm under the neck and shoulders, cradling the head. *Comments:*	☐	☐	☐	
14. Bend hips slightly. *Comments:*	☐	☐	☐	
15. On count of three, raise the patient's hips and back with the draw sheet. *Comments:*	☐	☐	☐	
16. Move the patient smoothly toward the head of bed. *Comments:*	☐	☐	☐	
17. Replace the pillow under the patient's head. *Comments:*	☐	☐	☐	
18. Tighten and tuck in the draw sheet. *Comments:*	☐	☐	☐	
19. Adjust the top bedding. *Comments:*	☐	☐	☐	
20. Carry out procedure completion actions. *Comments:*	☐	☐	☐	

Checklist for Procedure 17   Logrolling the Patient

Name _____ Date _____

School _____

Instructor _____

Course _____

Procedure 17 **Logrolling the Patient**	Able to Perform	Able to Perform with Assistance	Unable to Perform	Initials and Date
1. Carry out beginning procedure actions. *Comments:*	☐	☐	☐	
2. Ask for assistance. *Comments:*	☐	☐	☐	
3. Raise the bed to waist-high horizontal position and lock the wheels. *Comments:*	☐	☐	☐	
4. Lower the side rail on the side opposite to which the patient will be turned. *Comments:*	☐	☐	☐	
5. One assistant places hands under the patient's head and shoulders. *Comments:*	☐	☐	☐	
6. Second assistant places hands under the hips and legs. *Comments:*	☐	☐	☐	
7. Move the patient as a unit toward you. *Comments:*	☐	☐	☐	
8. Place a pillow lengthwise between the legs. *Comments:*	☐	☐	☐	
9. Fold the patient's arm over the chest. *Comments:*	☐	☐	☐	
10. Raise the side rail and check for security. *Comments:*	☐	☐	☐	

continued on the following page

continued from the previous page

Procedure 17	Able to Perform	Able to Perform with Assistance	Unable to Perform	Initials and Date
11. Go to the opposite side of the bed and lower the side rail. *Comments:*	☐	☐	☐	
12. Turn the patient on his side by using a turning sheet. *Comments:*	☐	☐	☐	
13. Reach over the patient and roll the turning sheet toward the patient. *Comments:*	☐	☐	☐	
14. If a turning sheet is not in position, position hands on the patient's far shoulder and hips. *Comments:*	☐	☐	☐	
15. Second assistant positions hands on the patient's far thigh and lower leg. *Comments:*	☐	☐	☐	
16. At signal, roll the patient toward both assistants in a single movement. *Comments:*	☐	☐	☐	
17. Place pillows behind the patient's back to maintain position. *Comments:*	☐	☐	☐	
18. Carry out procedure completion actions. *Comments:*	☐	☐	☐	

Checklist for Procedure 18   Applying a Transfer Belt

Name _____ Date _____

School _____

Instructor _____

Course _____

Procedure 18 Applying a Transfer Belt	Able to Perform	Able to Perform with Assistance	Unable to Perform	Initials and Date
1. Carry out beginning procedure actions. *Comments:*	☐	☐	☐	
2. Assemble equipment. *Comments:*	☐	☐	☐	
3. Explain the procedure. *Comments:*	☐	☐	☐	
4. Apply the belt over the patient's clothing. *Comments:*	☐	☐	☐	
5. Keep the belt at the patient's waist level. *Comments:*	☐	☐	☐	
6. Buckle the belt in front. *Comments:*	☐	☐	☐	
7. Check the fit of the belt by placing three fingers under it. *Comments:*	☐	☐	☐	
8. Check to ensure that the patient's feet are flat on the floor. *Comments:*	☐	☐	☐	
9. If using a wheelchair, keep the footrests out of the way. *Comments:*	☐	☐	☐	
10. Teach the patient to assist by pushing off with her hands when you count to three. *Comments:*	☐	☐	☐	

continued on the following page

continued from the previous page

Procedure 18	Able to Perform	Able to Perform with Assistance	Unable to Perform	Initials and Date
11. Grasp the belt using an underhand grasp. *Comments:*	☐	☐	☐	
12. Avoid overuse of the belt. *Comments:*	☐	☐	☐	
13. Bring the patient to a standing position and pivot to transfer. *Comments:*	☐	☐	☐	
14. Move the chair close enough so patient can feel it with her hands. *Comments:*	☐	☐	☐	
15. Remove the belt. *Comments:*	☐	☐	☐	
16. Carry out procedure completion actions. *Comments:*	☐	☐	☐	

Checklist for Procedure 19   Transferring the Patient from Bed to Chair—One Assistant

Name _____ Date _____

School _____

Instructor _____

Course _____

Procedure 19 Transferring the Patient from Bed to Chair— One Assistant	Able to Perform	Able to Perform with Assistance	Unable to Perform	Initials and Date
1. Carry out beginning procedure actions. *Comments:*	☐	☐	☐	
2. Assemble equipment. *Comments:*	☐	☐	☐	
3. Place chair so the patient moves toward her strong side. *Comments:*	☐	☐	☐	
4. Set the chair parallel with the bed. *Comments:*	☐	☐	☐	
5. If using wheelchair, lock the wheels and raise or remove the footrests. *Comments:*	☐	☐	☐	
6. Lock the bed wheels. *Comments:*	☐	☐	☐	
7. Stand against the right side of the bed with the side rail down. *Comments:*	☐	☐	☐	
8. Ask the patient to slide toward the right side of the bed. *Comments:*	☐	☐	☐	
9. Have the patient roll over onto her right side, flexing the knees and bending the right arm, to be used for propping the upper body. *Comments:*	☐	☐	☐	
10. Bend the elbow of the left arm to be used to push off from the bed. *Comments:*	☐	☐	☐	

continued on the following page

continued from the previous page

Procedure 19	Able to Perform	Able to Perform with Assistance	Unable to Perform	Initials and Date
11. Instruct the patient to use the elbow of her right arm to raise the upper body and push with the hand of the right arm so she comes to an upright position. *Comments:*	☐	☐	☐	
12. Instruct the patient to let her legs slide off the bed at the same time. *Comments:*	☐	☐	☐	
13. If the patient needs assistance, place one arm under her shoulders and one arm over and around her knees. *Comments:*	☐	☐	☐	
14. Raise the patient's upper body at the same time you move the legs off the bed. *Comments:*	☐	☐	☐	
15. Give the patient time to adjust to sitting up and then apply the transfer belt. *Comments:*	☐	☐	☐	
16. Assist the patient with putting on shoes and socks. *Comments:*	☐	☐	☐	
17. If the patient has a weak or paralyzed arm, provide support for it. *Comments:*	☐	☐	☐	
18. When the patient is ready to transfer, instruct her to move forward or closer to the edge of the mattress. *Comments:*	☐	☐	☐	
19. Instruct the patient to spread her knees, lean forward from the waist, and place her feet slightly back. *Comments:*	☐	☐	☐	
20. Spread your feet apart and bend your knees and hips, keeping your back straight. *Comments:*	☐	☐	☐	

Procedure 19	Able to Perform	Able to Perform with Assistance	Unable to Perform	Initials and Date
21. Hold the belt with an underhand grasp, one hand on each side of the front of the belt. *Comments:*	☐	☐	☐	
22. If the patient has a weak leg, press your knee against her knee or block the patient's foot with yours. *Comments:*	☐	☐	☐	
23. Tell the patient on the count of three to use her hands to press on the mattress, straighten her legs and knees, and come to a standing position. *Comments:*	☐	☐	☐	
24. If the patient cannot walk, have her pivot around to the front of the chair until the chair is touching the back of her legs. *Comments:*	☐	☐	☐	
25. Instruct the patient to place her hands on the arms of the chair, bend her knees, and then gently lower herself into the chair as you ease her downward. *Comments:*	☐	☐	☐	
26. Replace the footrests. *Comments:*	☐	☐	☐	
27. Position the patient comfortably. *Comments:*	☐	☐	☐	
28. Place the signal light within easy reach. *Comments:*	☐	☐	☐	
29. Straighten the bed and prepare it for the patient's return. *Comments:*	☐	☐	☐	
30. Carry out procedure completion actions. *Comments:*	☐	☐	☐	

Checklist for Procedure 20   Transferring the Patient from Bed to Chair—Two Assistants

Name _____ Date _____

School _____

Instructor _____

Course _____

Procedure 20 **Transferring the Patient from Bed to Chair—Two Assistants**	Able to Perform	Able to Perform with Assistance	Unable to Perform	Initials and Date
1. Follow steps 1 through 11 in Procedure 19. *Comments:*	☐	☐	☐	
2. Nursing assistants stand one on each side, facing the patient. *Comments:*	☐	☐	☐	
3. Each assistant places the hand closest to the patient through the belt, with an underhand grasp toward the front of the patient. Grasp the belt, toward the back, with the other hand. *Comments:*	☐	☐	☐	
4. The assistant closest to the chair stands with left leg farther back than the right, in a position to step or pivot around smoothly to allow the patient access to the chair. *Comments:*	☐	☐	☐	
5. Other assistant uses the left knee to brace the patient's weaker leg. *Comments:*	☐	☐	☐	
6. Instruct the patient to bend forward and place the palms of the hands on the edge of the mattress to push off. *Comments:*	☐	☐	☐	
7. The patient's knees should be spread apart, with both feet back and the stronger foot slightly in back of the weaker foot. *Comments:*	☐	☐	☐	
8. Both assistants should bend their knees to provide a broad base of support. *Comments:*	☐	☐	☐	

continued on the following page

continued from the previous page

Procedure 20	Able to Perform	Able to Perform with Assistance	Unable to Perform	Initials and Date
9. Ask the patient to stand on a count of three. *Comments:*	☐	☐	☐	
10. Allow the patient to stand for a moment and bear weight, keeping his head up. *Comments:*	☐	☐	☐	
11. Both assistants help the patient to pivot. *Comments:*	☐	☐	☐	
12. To sit, have the patient bend forward slightly, bend his knees, and lower onto the chair. Have him reach for the arms of the chair at the same time. *Comments:*	☐	☐	☐	
13. Position the patient comfortably. *Comments:*	☐	☐	☐	
14. Place the signal light within easy reach. *Comments:*	☐	☐	☐	
15. Straighten the bed and prepare it for the patient's return. *Comments:*	☐	☐	☐	
16. Carry out procedure completion actions. *Comments:*	☐	☐	☐	

Checklist for Procedure 21 Transferring the Patient from Chair to Bed—One Assistant

Name _____ Date _____

School _____

Instructor _____

Course _____

Procedure 21 Transferring the Patient from Chair to Bed—One Assistant	Able to Perform	Able to Perform with Assistance	Unable to Perform	Initials and Date
1. Carry out beginning procedure actions. *Comments:*	☐	☐	☐	
2. Assemble equipment: transfer belt. *Comments:*	☐	☐	☐	
3. Place the wheelchair so the patient moves toward his strongest side. *Comments:*	☐	☐	☐	
4. Set the wheelchair parallel with bed. *Comments:*	☐	☐	☐	
5. Place the bed in the lowest horizontal position and lock the wheels. *Comments:*	☐	☐	☐	
6. If necessary, fanfold top covers to the foot of the bed. *Comments:*	☐	☐	☐	
7. Raise the opposite side rail. *Comments:*	☐	☐	☐	
8. Lock the wheelchair and raise or remove the footrests. *Comments:*	☐	☐	☐	
9. Have the patient place both feet flat on the floor. *Comments:*	☐	☐	☐	
10. Place the transfer belt around the patient's waist. *Comments:*	☐	☐	☐	
11. Instruct the patient to move forward in the chair, to bend forward, and to spread his knees apart. Both feet should be back, with stronger foot slightly in back of the weaker foot. Both of the patient's arms should be on the arms of the chair. *Comments:*	☐	☐	☐	
12. Take hold of the transfer belt with an underhand grasp. *Comments:*	☐	☐	☐	

continued on the following page

continued from the previous page

Procedure 21	Able to Perform	Able to Perform with Assistance	Unable to Perform	Initials and Date
13. Use your knee or leg to brace the patient's weaker leg. *Comments:*	☐	☐	☐	
14. Ask the patient to push off the chair on the count of three and to stand. Provide assistance if necessary. *Comments:*	☐	☐	☐	
15. Allow the patient to remain standing for a time to stabilize position. *Comments:*	☐	☐	☐	
16. Keep your grasp on the transfer belt and continue to brace the weak leg if necessary. *Comments:*	☐	☐	☐	
17. Instruct the patient to step or pivot around to stand in front of the bed, facing away from it. *Comments:*	☐	☐	☐	
18. Tell the patient to sit when the edge of the mattress is touching the back of his legs. *Comments:*	☐	☐	☐	
19. Have the patient bend forward slightly, bend his knees, and lower himself onto the mattress. *Comments:*	☐	☐	☐	
20. When the patient is safely in bed, remove the transfer belt. *Comments:*	☐	☐	☐	
21. Remove the patient's slippers and robe. *Comments:*	☐	☐	☐	
22. Assist the patient with lying down, and position him as necessary. Draw top bedding over the patient. Fold the bath blanket (if used) from the wheelchair and return it to the bedside stand. *Comments:*	☐	☐	☐	
23. Make sure the call signal light is within reach. *Comments:*	☐	☐	☐	
24. Move the wheelchair out of the way. *Comments:*	☐	☐	☐	
25. Carry out procedure completion actions. *Comments:*	☐	☐	☐	

Checklist for Procedure 22 Transferring the Patient from Chair to Bed—Two Assistants

Name _____ Date _____

School _____

Instructor _____

Course _____

Procedure 22 **Transferring the Patient from Chair to Bed—Two Assistants**	Able to Perform	Able to Perform with Assistance	Unable to Perform	Initials and Date
1. Carry out beginning procedure actions. *Comments:*	☐	☐	☐	
2. Assemble equipment: transfer belt. *Comments:*	☐	☐	☐	
3. Place the wheelchair so patient moves toward her strongest side. *Comments:*	☐	☐	☐	
4. Set the wheelchair parallel with bed. *Comments:*	☐	☐	☐	
5. Place the bed in the lowest horizontal position and lock the wheels. *Comments:*	☐	☐	☐	
6. If necessary, fanfold top covers to the foot of the bed. *Comments:*	☐	☐	☐	
7. Raise the opposite side rail. *Comments:*	☐	☐	☐	
8. Lock the wheelchair and raise or remove the footrests. *Comments:*	☐	☐	☐	
9. Have the patient place both feet flat on the floor. *Comments:*	☐	☐	☐	
10. Place the transfer belt around patient's waist. *Comments:*	☐	☐	☐	

continued on the following page

continued from the previous page

Procedure 22	Able to Perform	Able to Perform with Assistance	Unable to Perform	Initials and Date
11. Instruct the patient to move forward in the chair, to bend forward, and to spread her knees apart. Both feet should be back, with stronger foot slightly in back of the weaker foot. Both of the patient's arms should be on the arms of the chair. *Comments:*	☐	☐	☐	
12. Each nursing assistant places the hand closest to the patient through the belt with an underhand grasp in front of the patient; the other hand goes toward the back. *Comments:*	☐	☐	☐	
13. The nursing assistant closest to the bed (on the patient's left side) stands in a position to step or pivot around smoothly to allow the patient access to the bed. This person should stand with the right leg further back than the left leg. *Comments:*	☐	☐	☐	
14. The other nursing assistant uses the left knee to brace the patient's weaker leg. *Comments:*	☐	☐	☐	
15. Ask the patient to push off the chair on the count of three and to stand. Provide assistance if necessary. *Comments:*	☐	☐	☐	
16. Allow the patient to remain standing for a time to stabilize position. *Comments:*	☐	☐	☐	
17. Keep your grasp on the transfer belt and continue to brace the weak leg if necessary. *Comments:*	☐	☐	☐	
18. Instruct the patient to step or pivot around to stand in front of the bed, facing away from it. *Comments:*	☐	☐	☐	
19. Tell the patient to sit when the edge of the mattress is touching the back of her legs. *Comments:*	☐	☐	☐	

Procedure 22	Able to Perform	Able to Perform with Assistance	Unable to Perform	Initials and Date
20. Have the patient bend forward slightly, bend her knees, and lower herself onto the mattress. *Comments:*	☐	☐	☐	
21. When the patient is safely in bed, remove the transfer belt. *Comments:*	☐	☐	☐	
22. Remove the patient's slippers and robe. *Comments:*	☐	☐	☐	
23. Assist the patient to lie down, and position her as necessary. Draw top bedding over the patient. Fold the bath blanket (if used) from the wheelchair and return it to the bedside stand. *Comments:*	☐	☐	☐	
24. Make sure the call signal light is within reach. *Comments:*	☐	☐	☐	
25. Move the wheelchair out of the way. *Comments:*	☐	☐	☐	
26. Carry out procedure completion actions. *Comments:*	☐	☐	☐	

Checklist for Procedure 23   Independent Transfer, Standby Assist

Name _____ Date _____

School _____

Instructor _____

Course _____

Procedure 23 **Independent Transfer, Standby Assist**	Able to Perform	Able to Perform with Assistance	Unable to Perform	Initials and Date
1. Carry out beginning procedure actions. *Comments:*	☐	☐	☐	
2. Assemble equipment. *Comments:*	☐	☐	☐	
3. Place the wheelchair so patient moves toward his strong side. *Comments:*	☐	☐	☐	
4. Set the wheelchair parallel with the bed. *Comments:*	☐	☐	☐	
5. Lock the wheelchair and raise or remove the footrests. *Comments:*	☐	☐	☐	
6. Lock the bed wheels. *Comments:*	☐	☐	☐	
7. Stand against the right side of bed with the side rail down. *Comments:*	☐	☐	☐	
8. Ask the patient to slide toward the right side of the bed. *Comments:*	☐	☐	☐	
9. Have the patient roll over onto his right side, flexing the knees and bending the right arm, to be used for propping the upper body. *Comments:*	☐	☐	☐	
10. Bend the elbow of the left arm to be used to push off from the bed. *Comments:*	☐	☐	☐	

continued on the following page

continued from the previous page

Procedure 23	Able to Perform	Able to Perform with Assistance	Unable to Perform	Initials and Date
11. Instruct the patient to use the elbow of his right arm to raise the upper body and push with the hand of the right arm so he comes to an upright position. *Comments:*	☐	☐	☐	
12. Instruct the patient to let his legs slide off the bed at the same time. *Comments:*	☐	☐	☐	
13. If the patient needs assistance, place one arm under his shoulders and one arm over and around his knees. *Comments:*	☐	☐	☐	
14. Raise the patient's upper body at the same time you move the legs off the bed. *Comments:*	☐	☐	☐	
15. Give the patient time to adjust to sitting up and then apply the transfer belt. *Comments:*	☐	☐	☐	
16. Assist the patient with putting on shoes and socks. *Comments:*	☐	☐	☐	
17. If the patient has a weak or paralyzed arm, provide support for it. *Comments:*	☐	☐	☐	
18. When the patient is ready to transfer, instruct him to move forward or closer to the edge of the mattress. *Comments:*	☐	☐	☐	
19. Have the patient place the strongest foot slightly in back of the other foot. The patient's knees should be slightly apart. *Comments:*	☐	☐	☐	
20. Instruct the patient to place the palms of the hands at the edge of the bed and to lean slightly forward. *Comments:*	☐	☐	☐	

Procedure 23	Able to Perform	Able to Perform with Assistance	Unable to Perform	Initials and Date
21. Tell the patient to press his hands into the bed to push off and assume a standing position. *Comments:*	☐	☐	☐	
22. Once standing, have the patient reach for the far arm of the chair and then step or pivot to stand in front of the chair. *Comments:*	☐	☐	☐	
23. Instruct the patient to sit when the edge of the chair is felt against the back of the legs. *Comments:*	☐	☐	☐	
24. Carry out procedure completion actions. *Comments:*	☐	☐	☐	
25. Reverse these directions when transferring from the chair to bed. *Comments:*	☐	☐	☐	

Checklist for Procedure 24   Transferring the Patient from Bed to Stretcher

Name _____ Date _____

School _____

Instructor _____

Course _____

Procedure 24 **Transferring the Patient from Bed to Stretcher**	Able to Perform	Able to Perform with Assistance	Unable to Perform	Initials and Date
1. Carry out beginning procedure actions. *Comments:*	☐	☐	☐	
2. Assemble equipment. *Comments:*	☐	☐	☐	
3. Lock the wheels of the bed. *Comments:*	☐	☐	☐	
4. Raise the bed to a horizontal position equal to the height of the stretcher. *Comments:*	☐	☐	☐	
5. Lower the side rails. *Comments:*	☐	☐	☐	
6. Place a bath blanket over the patient. *Comments:*	☐	☐	☐	
7. Fanfold top covers to the foot of the bed. *Comments:*	☐	☐	☐	
8. Roll the turning sheet up against the patient on both sides. *Comments:*	☐	☐	☐	
9. Position the stretcher close to the bed and lock the wheels. *Comments:*	☐	☐	☐	
10. Have two or three people stand along the open side of the stretcher. *Comments:*	☐	☐	☐	

continued on the following page

continued from the previous page

Procedure 24	Able to Perform	Able to Perform with Assistance	Unable to Perform	Initials and Date
11. One assistant stands on the open side of the bed. *Comments:*	☐	☐	☐	
12. The assistant at the end of the bed grasps the moving sheet, with an overhand grasp, placing one hand by the patient's legs and the other by the hips. *Comments:*	☐	☐	☐	
13. The middle assistant grasps the moving sheet, with an overhand grasp, placing one hand by the patient's hips and the other by the shoulders. *Comments:*	☐	☐	☐	
14. The assistant at the head of the bed grasps the turning sheet, with an overhand grasp, placing one hand by the patient's shoulder and head. *Comments:*	☐	☐	☐	
15. On the count of three, all persons slide the moving sheet from bed to stretcher. *Comments:*	☐	☐	☐	
16. Center the patient on the stretcher in good body alignment. *Comments:*	☐	☐	☐	
17. Secure the stretcher safety belt. *Comments:*	☐	☐	☐	
18. Raise the side rails of the stretcher. *Comments:*	☐	☐	☐	
19. Transport the patient as directed. *Comments:*	☐	☐	☐	
20. Prepare the bed for the patient's return. *Comments:*	☐	☐	☐	
21. Carry out procedure completion actions. *Comments:*	☐	☐	☐	

Checklist for Procedure 25   Transferring the Patient from Stretcher to Bed

Name _____ Date _____

School _____

Instructor _____

Course _____

Procedure 25 Transferring the Patient from Stretcher to Bed	Able to Perform	Able to Perform with Assistance	Unable to Perform	Initials and Date
1. Carry out beginning procedure actions. *Comments:*	☐	☐	☐	
2. Assemble equipment. *Comments:*	☐	☐	☐	
3. Lock the wheels of the bed. *Comments:*	☐	☐	☐	
4. Raise the bed to a horizontal position equal to the height of the stretcher. *Comments:*	☐	☐	☐	
5. Lower the side rails. *Comments:*	☐	☐	☐	
6. Fanfold top covers to the foot of the bed. *Comments:*	☐	☐	☐	
7. Place a bath blanket over the patient. *Comments:*	☐	☐	☐	
8. Roll the turning sheet up against the patient on both sides. *Comments:*	☐	☐	☐	
9. Position the stretcher close to the bed and lock the wheels. *Comments:*	☐	☐	☐	
10. Lower the side rails of the stretcher. *Comments:*	☐	☐	☐	

continued on the following page

continued from the previous page

Procedure 25	Able to Perform	Able to Perform with Assistance	Unable to Perform	Initials and Date
11. One assistant stands along the open side of the stretcher. *Comments:*	☐	☐	☐	
12. Have two or three people stand on the open side of the bed. *Comments:*	☐	☐	☐	
13. The assistant at the end of the bed grasps the moving sheet, with an overhand grasp, placing one hand by the patient's legs and the other by the hips. *Comments:*	☐	☐	☐	
14. The middle assistant grasps the moving sheet, with an overhand grasp, placing one hand by the patient's hips and the other by the shoulders. *Comments:*	☐	☐	☐	
15. The assistant at the head of the bed grasps the turning sheet, with an overhand grasp, placing one hand by the patient's shoulder and head. *Comments:*	☐	☐	☐	
16. On the count of three, all persons slide the moving sheet from stretcher to bed. *Comments:*	☐	☐	☐	
17. Center the patient on the bed in good body alignment. *Comments:*	☐	☐	☐	
18. Properly position the patient. *Comments:*	☐	☐	☐	
19. Raise the side rails of the bed, if ordered. *Comments:*	☐	☐	☐	
20. Carry out procedure completion actions. *Comments:*	☐	☐	☐	

Checklist for Procedure 26   Transferring the Patient with a Mechanical Lift

Name _____ Date _____

School _____

Instructor _____

Course _____

Procedure 26 **Transferring the Patient with a Mechanical Lift**	Able to Perform	Able to Perform with Assistance	Unable to Perform	Initials and Date
1. Carry out beginning procedure actions. *Comments:*	☐	☐	☐	
2. Assemble equipment. *Comments:*	☐	☐	☐	
3. Place a wheelchair or other chair parallel to the foot of the bed, facing the head. *Comments:*	☐	☐	☐	
4. Lock the wheelchair, if used. *Comments:*	☐	☐	☐	
5. Elevate the bed to a comfortable working height. *Comments:*	☐	☐	☐	
6. Lock the bed wheels. *Comments:*	☐	☐	☐	
7. Lower the nearest side rail. *Comments:*	☐	☐	☐	
8. Roll the patient toward you. *Comments:*	☐	☐	☐	
9. Position the sling beneath the patient's body behind shoulder, thighs, and buttocks. *Comments:*	☐	☐	☐	
10. Check to be sure sling is smooth. *Comments:*	☐	☐	☐	

continued on the following page

continued from the previous page

Procedure 26	Able to Perform	Able to Perform with Assistance	Unable to Perform	Initials and Date
11. Roll the patient back onto the sling and position properly. *Comments:*	☐	☐	☐	
12. If the sling has inserts for metal bars, insert them now. *Comments:*	☐	☐	☐	
13. Position the lift frame over the bed. *Comments:*	☐	☐	☐	
14. Lock the lift legs. *Comments:*	☐	☐	☐	
15. Attach suspension straps or chains to the sling and check fasteners for security. *Comments:*	☐	☐	☐	
16. Position the patient's crossed arms inside the straps. *Comments:*	☐	☐	☐	
17. Secure the straps or chains if necessary. *Comments:*	☐	☐	☐	
18. One assistant operates the lift and the other assistant guides the movement of the patient. *Comments:*	☐	☐	☐	
19. Lock the hydraulic mechanism. *Comments:*	☐	☐	☐	
20. Slowly raise the boom of the lift until the patient is suspended over the bed. *Comments:*	☐	☐	☐	
21. Talk to the patient while slowly lifting him free of the bed. *Comments:*	☐	☐	☐	
22. Guide the lift away from the bed. *Comments:*	☐	☐	☐	

Procedure 26	Able to Perform	Able to Perform with Assistance	Unable to Perform	Initials and Date
23. Position the patient and lift over the chair or wheelchair. *Comments:*	☐	☐	☐	
24. Slowly lower the patient into the chair or wheelchair. *Comments:*	☐	☐	☐	
25. Check position of the patient's feet and hands. *Comments:*	☐	☐	☐	
26. One assistant stands behind the chair to pull and guide the patient's hips back into position. *Comments:*	☐	☐	☐	
27. Unhook the suspension straps or chains and remove the lift. *Comments:*	☐	☐	☐	
28. Position the footrests to support the feet. *Comments:*	☐	☐	☐	
29. If the patient is in a chair, the sling can remain underneath the patient for transfer back to bed. *Comments:*	☐	☐	☐	
30. If the sling has metal bars, remove them and make sure the sling is smooth and wrinkle-free. *Comments:*	☐	☐	☐	
31. Place the signal light within reach. *Comments:*	☐	☐	☐	
32. When the patient is transferred back into bed, remove the sling. *Comments:*	☐	☐	☐	
33. Pull top covers up and position the patient. *Comments:*	☐	☐	☐	

continued on the following page

continued from the previous page

Procedure 26	Able to Perform	Able to Perform with Assistance	Unable to Perform	Initials and Date
34. Raise the side rails, if necessary. *Comments:*	☐	☐	☐	
35. Place the signal light within reach. *Comments:*	☐	☐	☐	
36. Carry out procedure completion actions. *Comments:*	☐	☐	☐	

Checklist for Procedure 27   Transferring the Patient onto and off the Toilet

Name _____ Date _____

School _____

Instructor _____

Course _____

Procedure 27 Transferring the Patient onto and off the Toilet	Able to Perform	Able to Perform with Assistance	Unable to Perform	Initials and Date
1. Carry out beginning procedure actions. *Comments:*	☐	☐	☐	
2. Assemble equipment. *Comments:*	☐	☐	☐	
3. Position the wheelchair at a right angle to the toilet or commode to face the wall rail. *Comments:*	☐	☐	☐	
4. Lock the wheels. *Comments:*	☐	☐	☐	
5. Raise or remove the footrests. *Comments:*	☐	☐	☐	
6. Place a transfer belt around the patient's waist. *Comments:*	☐	☐	☐	
7. Use an underhand grasp with one hand toward the patient's back and the other hand toward the patient's front. *Comments:*	☐	☐	☐	
8. Instruct the patient to lean forward slightly, placing the strongest foot slightly behind the other foot, and to bring herself to a standing position. *Comments:*	☐	☐	☐	
9. Have the patient grasp the wall rail with both hands. *Comments:*	☐	☐	☐	
10. Have the patient pivot or step around until she feels the toilet against the back of her legs. *Comments:*	☐	☐	☐	
11. Slide the pants and underwear down over the patient's knees. *Comments:*	☐	☐	☐	

continued on the following page

continued from the previous page

Procedure 27	Able to Perform	Able to Perform with Assistance	Unable to Perform	Initials and Date
12. Assist the patient to a sitting position on the toilet. *Comments:*	☐	☐	☐	
13. Allow her time to eliminate. *Comments:*	☐	☐	☐	
14. When the patient is finished, put on disposable gloves. *Comments:*	☐	☐	☐	
15. Instruct the patient to stand and reach for the wall rail. *Comments:*	☐	☐	☐	
16. Use toilet tissue to clean the patient, if she is unable to do this herself. *Comments:*	☐	☐	☐	
17. If the patient is steady, remove and dispose of your gloves. *Comments:*	☐	☐	☐	
18. Pull the patient's pants or underwear up. *Comments:*	☐	☐	☐	
19. If sink is close enough, ask the patient to pivot or step to the sink to wash her hands before sitting in the wheelchair. *Comments:*	☐	☐	☐	
20. If a sink is not close, have the patient sit in the wheelchair. *Comments:*	☐	☐	☐	
21. Unlock the wheels, replace the footrests, and move the wheelchair to the sink so the patient can wash her hands. *Comments:*	☐	☐	☐	
22. Wash your hands. *Comments:*	☐	☐	☐	
23. Assist the patient to leave the bathroom. *Comments:*	☐	☐	☐	
24. Make sure the patient is comfortable and the signal light is within reach. *Comments:*	☐	☐	☐	
25. Carry out procedure completion actions. *Comments:*	☐	☐	☐	

Checklist for Procedure 28 Transferring the Patient into and out of the Tub

Name _____ Date _____

School _____

Instructor _____

Course _____

Procedure 28 Transferring the Patient into and out of the Tub	Able to Perform	Able to Perform with Assistance	Unable to Perform	Initials and Date
1. Carry out beginning procedure actions. *Comments:*	☐	☐	☐	
2. Assemble equipment. *Comments:*	☐	☐	☐	
3. Place a sturdy chair beside the tub, facing the faucets. *Comments:*	☐	☐	☐	
4. Have the patient transfer from wheelchair to chair and then into the tub and onto the tub chair. *Comments:*	☐	☐	☐	
5. Instruct the patient to place the leg closest to the tub into the tub. *Comments:*	☐	☐	☐	
6. Tell the patient to use the strongest arm to reach for the wall rail. *Comments:*	☐	☐	☐	
7. As the patient slides onto the tub chair, have her bring the other leg over the side of the tub. *Comments:*	☐	☐	☐	
8. Have the patient proceed with her bath, giving assistance as needed. *Comments:*	☐	☐	☐	
9. If possible, provide privacy while staying within hearing distance. *Comments:*	☐	☐	☐	

continued on the following page

continued from the previous page

Procedure 28	Able to Perform	Able to Perform with Assistance	Unable to Perform	Initials and Date
10. When the patient is finished with her bath, she should get the strong leg out of the tub and use the strong arm to move herself onto the chair. *Comments:*	☐	☐	☐	
11. Instruct her to use the strong arm to move her weaker leg out of the tub. *Comments:*	☐	☐	☐	
12. Assist the patient to dry and dress if necessary. *Comments:*	☐	☐	☐	
13. Carry out procedure completion actions. *Comments:*	☐	☐	☐	
14. Disinfect the tub and tub chair. *Comments:*	☐	☐	☐	

Checklist for Procedure 29   Transferring a Patient into and out of a Car

Name _____ Date _____

School _____

Instructor _____

Course _____

Procedure 29 Transferring a Patient into and out of a Car	Able to Perform	Able to Perform with Assistance	Unable to Perform	Initials and Date
1. Carry out beginning procedure actions. *Comments:*	☐	☐	☐	
2. Assemble equipment. *Comments:*	☐	☐	☐	
3. Place the wheelchair at a 45° angle to the car, with brakes set. *Comments:*	☐	☐	☐	
4. If necessary, place a transfer belt on the patient. *Comments:*	☐	☐	☐	
5. Have the patient come to a standing position. *Comments:*	☐	☐	☐	
6. If transferring to the stronger side, the dashboard and car door can be used for support. If moving toward the weaker side, instruct the patient to use the strong arm and the door with the window open for support. *Comments:*	☐	☐	☐	
7. Have another person hold the door for stability. *Comments:*	☐	☐	☐	
8. Instruct the patient to pivot or step around so the side of the car seat is touching the back of the legs. *Comments:*	☐	☐	☐	
9. After she sits down, have the patient raise one leg at a time into the car to face forward. *Comments:*	☐	☐	☐	

continued on the following page

continued from the previous page

Procedure 29	Able to Perform	Able to Perform with Assistance	Unable to Perform	Initials and Date
10. Assist with the seat belt. *Comments:*	☐	☐	☐	
11. Reverse the procedure to assist the patient out of the car. *Comments:*	☐	☐	☐	
12. Carry out procedure completion actions. *Comments:*	☐	☐	☐	

Checklist for Procedure 30   Assisting the Patient to Walk with a Cane and Three-Point Gait

Name _____ Date _____

School _____

Instructor _____

Course _____

Procedure 30 Assisting the Patient to Walk with a Cane and Three-Point Gait	Able to Perform	Able to Perform with Assistance	Unable to Perform	Initials and Date
1. Carry out beginning procedure actions. *Comments:*	☐	☐	☐	
2. Assemble equipment. *Comments:*	☐	☐	☐	
3. Make sure patient has on sturdy shoes with nonskid soles. Check that clothing does not hang down over shoes. *Comments:*	☐	☐	☐	
4. Place the bed in the lowest horizontal position with brakes locked. *Comments:*	☐	☐	☐	
5. Assist the patient to sit on the edge of the bed. *Comments:*	☐	☐	☐	
6. Place a gait belt on the patient and assist him to a standing position. *Comments:*	☐	☐	☐	
7. Stand on the patient's affected side. Place your closest hand in the gait belt, using an underhand grasp. *Comments:*	☐	☐	☐	
8. Instruct the patient to hold the cane on his stronger side, with the tip about 4 inches to the side of the stronger foot. *Comments:*	☐	☐	☐	
9. Have the patient to shift his body weight to the strong leg and advance the cane about 4 inches supporting his weight on the strong leg and the cane. *Comments:*	☐	☐	☐	

continued on the following page

continued from the previous page

Procedure 30	Able to Perform	Able to Perform with Assistance	Unable to Perform	Initials and Date
10. Instruct the patient to move the weak leg forward so it is even with the cane. *Comments:*	☐	☐	☐	
11. Have the patient shift his weight to the weak leg and the cane, moving the strong leg forward, ahead of the cane. This pattern is repeated while the patient is walking. *Comments:*	☐	☐	☐	
12. Note the patient's endurance, balance, and strength while walking. *Comments:*	☐	☐	☐	
13. Stop immediately if the patient has trouble and help him to the closest chair. Call the nurse. *Comments:*	☐	☐	☐	
14. Assist the patient to sit in the chair or to lie down in bed. *Comments:*	☐	☐	☐	
15. Remove the gait belt. *Comments:*	☐	☐	☐	
16. Store the cane in an appropriate area. *Comments:*	☐	☐	☐	
17. Document the distance the patient ambulated and his tolerance of the procedure. *Comments:*	☐	☐	☐	
18. Carry out procedure completion actions. *Comments:*	☐	☐	☐	

Checklist for Procedure 31   Assisting the Patient to Walk with a Walker and Three-Point Gait

Name _____ Date _____

School _____

Instructor _____

Course _____

Procedure 31 **Assisting the Patient to Walk with a Walker and Three-Point Gait**	Able to Perform	Able to Perform with Assistance	Unable to Perform	Initials and Date
1. Carry out beginning procedure actions. *Comments:*	☐	☐	☐	
2. Assemble equipment. *Comments:*	☐	☐	☐	
3. Make sure the patient has on sturdy shoes with nonskid soles. Check that clothing does not hang down over her shoes. *Comments:*	☐	☐	☐	
4. Place a gait belt on the patient and assist her to a standing position. *Comments:*	☐	☐	☐	
5. Place the walker in front of the patient and have her grasp the walker with both hands. Stand on the patient's affected side. *Comments:*	☐	☐	☐	
6. Place your closest hand in the gait belt, using an underhand grasp. *Comments:*	☐	☐	☐	
7. Instruct the patient to stand with her weight evenly distributed between the walker and both legs, with the walker in front of her. *Comments:*	☐	☐	☐	
8. Have the patient shift her weight to the strong leg as she lifts and moves the walker 6 to 8 inches ahead. *Comments:*	☐	☐	☐	

continued on the following page

continued from the previous page

Procedure 31	Able to Perform	Able to Perform with Assistance	Unable to Perform	Initials and Date
9. The patient should then bring her weak foot forward into the walker. *Comments:*	☐	☐	☐	
10. Instruct her to bring her strong foot forward even with the weak foot. *Comments:*	☐	☐	☐	
11. This process is repeated while the patient is walking. *Comments:*	☐	☐	☐	
12. Note the patient's endurance, balance, and strength while walking. *Comments:*	☐	☐	☐	
13. Stop immediately if the patient has trouble and help her to the closest chair. Call the nurse. *Comments:*	☐	☐	☐	
14. Assist the patient to sit in the chair or to lie down in bed. *Comments:*	☐	☐	☐	
15. Remove the gait belt. *Comments:*	☐	☐	☐	
16. Store the walker in an appropriate area. *Comments:*	☐	☐	☐	
17. Document the distance the patient ambulated and her tolerance of the procedure. *Comments:*	☐	☐	☐	
18. Carry out procedure completion actions. *Comments:*	☐	☐	☐	

Checklist for Procedure 32   Assisting the Falling Patient

Name _____ Date _____

School _____

Instructor _____

Course _____

Procedure 32 **Assisting the Falling Patient**	Able to Perform	Able to Perform with Assistance	Unable to Perform	Initials and Date
1. Keep your back straight; bend from the hips and knees. Maintain a broad base of support as you assist the falling patient. *Comments:*	☐	☐	☐	
2. Maintain your grasp on the transfer belt. *Comments:*	☐	☐	☐	
3. Ease the patient to the floor, protecting her head. *Comments:*	☐	☐	☐	
4. As you ease the patient to the floor, bend your knees and go down with the patient. *Comments:*	☐	☐	☐	
5. Call for help. *Comments:*	☐	☐	☐	
6. Assist in returning the patient to the bed or chair. *Comments:*	☐	☐	☐	
7. Carry out procedure completion actions. *Comments:*	☐	☐	☐	

Checklist for Procedure 33 Measuring an Oral Temperature (Glass Thermometer)

Name _____ Date _____

School _____

Instructor _____

Course _____

Procedure 33 **Measuring an Oral Temperature (Glass Thermometer)**	Able to Perform	Able to Perform with Assistance	Unable to Perform	Initials and Date
1. Carry out beginning procedure actions. *Comments:*	☐	☐	☐	
2. Assemble equipment. *Comments:*	☐	☐	☐	
3. Have the patient rest in a comfortable position in a bed or chair. *Comments:*	☐	☐	☐	
4. If the patient has had anything to eat or drink or has smoked, wait 15 minutes before taking an oral temperature. *Comments:*	☐	☐	☐	
5. Apply disposable gloves. *Comments:*	☐	☐	☐	
6. Remove the thermometer from the container by holding the stem end. *Comments:*	☐	☐	☐	
7. Rinse the thermometer with cold water and wipe with tissue from stem to bulb end if it has been in disinfectant. *Comments:*	☐	☐	☐	
8. Check to ensure the thermometer is intact. *Comments:*	☐	☐	☐	
9. Read the center column. It should register below 96°F. If necessary, shake it down. *Comments:*	☐	☐	☐	
10. To shake down, move away from tables and other hard objects. Grasp the stem tightly between your thumb and fingers. Shake down with a downward motion. *Comments:*	☐	☐	☐	

continued on the following page

continued from the previous page

Procedure 33	Able to Perform	Able to Perform with Assistance	Unable to Perform	Initials and Date
11. If used by your facility, place the thermometer in a disposable plastic cover sheath. *Comments:*	☐	☐	☐	
12. Insert the bulb end of the thermometer under the patient's tongue, toward the side of the mouth. *Comments:*	☐	☐	☐	
13. Tell the patient to hold the thermometer gently with lips closed for 3 minutes. *Comments:*	☐	☐	☐	
14. Remove the thermometer, holding it by the stem. *Comments:*	☐	☐	☐	
15. Wipe from stem end toward bulb end. *Comments:*	☐	☐	☐	
16. Discard tissue in the proper container. *Comments:*	☐	☐	☐	
17. Read the thermometer and record the temperature on a notepad. *Comments:*	☐	☐	☐	
18. Place the thermometer in the container for used thermometers. *Comments:*	☐	☐	☐	
19. If the thermometer is to be reused for this patient: wash it twice in cold water and soap with two cotton balls, wiping from stem to bulb. Rinse and dry it. Return it to the individual disinfectant-filled holder. *Comments:*	☐	☐	☐	
20. Remove gloves and discard according to facility policy. *Comments:*	☐	☐	☐	
21. Carry out procedure completion actions. *Comments:*	☐	☐	☐	
22. Report any unusual variations to the nurse at once. *Comments:*	☐	☐	☐	

Checklist for Procedure 34   Measuring Temperature Using a Sheath-Covered Thermometer

Name _____   Date _____

School _____

Instructor _____

Course _____

Procedure 34 **Measuring Temperature Using a Sheath-Covered Thermometer**	Able to Perform	Able to Perform with Assistance	Unable to Perform	Initials and Date
1. Carry out beginning procedure actions. *Comments:*	☐	☐	☐	
2. Assemble equipment. *Comments:*	☐	☐	☐	
3. Have the patient rest in a comfortable position in a bed or chair. *Comments:*	☐	☐	☐	
4. If the patient has had anything to eat or drink or has smoked, wait 15 minutes before taking an oral temperature. *Comments:*	☐	☐	☐	
5. Apply disposable gloves. *Comments:*	☐	☐	☐	
6. Shake the thermometer down to below 96°F. *Comments:*	☐	☐	☐	
7. Insert thermometer into the marked end of a protective sheath wrapper. *Comments:*	☐	☐	☐	
8. Peel back the outer paper cover to expose the inner plastic sheath. *Comments:*	☐	☐	☐	
9. Grasp the outer paper wrapper. *Comments:*	☐	☐	☐	

continued on the following page

continued from the previous page

Procedure 34	Able to Perform	Able to Perform with Assistance	Unable to Perform	Initials and Date
10. Twist the paper wrapper to break the seal with the tab and remove the outer paper wrapper. *Comments:*	☐	☐	☐	
11. Keeping the plastic sheath over the thermometer, insert the bulb end of the thermometer under the patient's tongue, toward the side of the mouth. *Comments:*	☐	☐	☐	
12. Tell the patient to hold the thermometer gently with the lips closed for 3 minutes. *Comments:*	☐	☐	☐	
13. Remove the thermometer and discard the plastic sheath. *Comments:*	☐	☐	☐	
14. Read and shake down. *Comments:*	☐	☐	☐	
15. Record the temperature on a notepad. *Comments:*	☐	☐	☐	
16. Use a new sheath each time the thermometer is reused. *Comments:*	☐	☐	☐	
17. Remove gloves and discard according to facility policy. *Comments:*	☐	☐	☐	
18. Carry out procedure completion actions. *Comments:*	☐	☐	☐	
19. Report any unusual variations to the nurse at once. *Comments:*	☐	☐	☐	

Checklist for Procedure 35 Measuring a Rectal Temperature (Glass Thermometer)

Name _____ Date _____

School _____

Instructor _____

Course _____

Procedure 35 **Measuring a Rectal Temperature** **(Glass Thermometer)**	Able to Perform	Able to Perform with Assistance	Unable to Perform	Initials and Date
1. Carry out beginning procedure actions. *Comments:*	☐	☐	☐	
2. Assemble equipment. *Comments:*	☐	☐	☐	
3. Put up the opposite side rail. *Comments:*	☐	☐	☐	
4. Lower the back rest of the bed. *Comments:*	☐	☐	☐	
5. Ask the patient to turn to the left side; assist if needed. *Comments:*	☐	☐	☐	
6. Place a small amount of lubricant on a tissue. *Comments:*	☐	☐	☐	
7. Apply disposable gloves. *Comments:*	☐	☐	☐	
8. Remove the thermometer and shake down to below 96°F. *Comments:*	☐	☐	☐	
9. Check to ensure the thermometer is intact. *Comments:*	☐	☐	☐	
10. Apply a small amount of the lubricant to the bulb with a tissue. *Comments:*	☐	☐	☐	
11. Fold the top bedclothes back to expose the patient's anal area. *Comments:*	☐	☐	☐	

continued on the following page

continued from the previous page

Procedure 35	Able to Perform	Able to Perform with Assistance	Unable to Perform	Initials and Date
12. Separate the buttocks with one hand. *Comments:*	☐	☐	☐	
13. Insert the thermometer gently 1 inch into the rectum and hold in place. *Comments:*	☐	☐	☐	
14. Replace the bedclothes for privacy. *Comments:*	☐	☐	☐	
15. Hold the thermometer in place for 3 to 5 minutes. *Comments:*	☐	☐	☐	
16. Remove the thermometer. *Comments:*	☐	☐	☐	
17. Wipe from stem toward the bulb end and discard the tissue. *Comments:*	☐	☐	☐	
18. Read the thermometer and record the reading on a pad. *Comments:*	☐	☐	☐	
19. Wipe the lubricant from the patient and discard the tissue. *Comments:*	☐	☐	☐	
20. Place the thermometer in the container for used thermometers. *Comments:*	☐	☐	☐	
21. If the thermometer is to be reused for this patient: wash it twice in cold water and soap with two cotton balls, wiping from stem to bulb. Rinse and dry it. Return it to the individual disinfectant-filled holder. *Comments:*	☐	☐	☐	
22. Remove gloves and discard according to facility policy. *Comments:*	☐	☐	☐	
23. Lower the opposite side rail. *Comments:*	☐	☐	☐	
24. Carry out procedure completion actions. *Comments:*	☐	☐	☐	

Checklist for Procedure 36 Measuring an Axillary or Groin Temperature (Glass Thermometer)

Name _____ Date _____

School _____

Instructor _____

Course _____

Procedure 36 **Measuring an Axillary or Groin Temperature (Glass Thermometer)**	Able to Perform	Able to Perform with Assistance	Unable to Perform	Initials and Date
1. Carry out beginning procedure actions. *Comments:*	☐	☐	☐	
2. Assemble equipment. *Comments:*	☐	☐	☐	
3. Remove the thermometer and shake down to below 96°F. *Comments:*	☐	☐	☐	
4. Cover the thermometer with a disposable sheath, if used. *Comments:*	☐	☐	☐	
5. Apply gloves if the groin area is to be used. *Comments:*	☐	☐	☐	
6. Wipe the area dry and place the thermometer. *Comments:*	☐	☐	☐	
7. When using the axillary site, hold the patient's arm close to the body. *Comments:*	☐	☐	☐	
8. When using the groin area, the thermometer must be in the fold against the body. *Comments:*	☐	☐	☐	
9. Hold the thermometer in place for 10 minutes. *Comments:*	☐	☐	☐	
10. Remove, wipe, and discard sheath if used. *Comments:*	☐	☐	☐	

continued on the following page

continued from the previous page

Procedure 36	Able to Perform	Able to Perform with Assistance	Unable to Perform	Initials and Date
11. Read the thermometer and record the reading on a notepad. *Comments:*	☐	☐	☐	
12. Shake the thermometer down. *Comments:*	☐	☐	☐	
13. If the thermometer is to be reused for this patient: wash it twice in cold water and soap with two cotton balls, wiping from stem to bulb. Rinse and dry it. Return it to the individual disinfectant-filled holder. *Comments:*	☐	☐	☐	
14. If used, remove and discard gloves. *Comments:*	☐	☐	☐	
15. Carry out procedure completion actions. *Comments:*	☐	☐	☐	

Checklist for Procedure 37   Measuring an Oral Temperature (Electronic Thermometer)

Name _____ Date _____

School _____

Instructor _____

Course _____

Procedure 37 **Measuring an Oral Temperature (Electronic Thermometer)**	Able to Perform	Able to Perform with Assistance	Unable to Perform	Initials and Date
1. Carry out beginning procedure actions. *Comments:*	☐	☐	☐	
2. Assemble equipment. *Comments:*	☐	☐	☐	
3. If the patient has had anything to eat or drink or has smoked, wait 15 minutes before taking an oral temperature. *Comments:*	☐	☐	☐	
4. Apply gloves if it is your facility's policy. *Comments:*	☐	☐	☐	
5. Cover the probe with a protective sheath. *Comments:*	☐	☐	☐	
6. Insert the covered probe under the patient's tongue toward the side of the mouth. *Comments:*	☐	☐	☐	
7. Hold the probe in place. *Comments:*	☐	☐	☐	
8. Instruct the patient to close his mouth and breathe through his nose. *Comments:*	☐	☐	☐	
9. Remove the probe when the buzzer signals that the temperature has been determined. *Comments:*	☐	☐	☐	

continued on the following page

continued from the previous page

Procedure 37	Able to Perform	Able to Perform with Assistance	Unable to Perform	Initials and Date
10. Discard the sheath. *Comments:*	☐	☐	☐	
11. Remove gloves, if worn. *Comments:*	☐	☐	☐	
12. Return the probe to its proper position. *Comments:*	☐	☐	☐	
13. Record the temperature on a notepad. *Comments:*	☐	☐	☐	
14. Return the thermometer unit to the charger. *Comments:*	☐	☐	☐	
15. Carry out procedure completion actions. *Comments:*	☐	☐	☐	

Checklist for Procedure 38   Measuring a Rectal Temperature (Electronic Thermometer)

Name _____ Date _____

School _____

Instructor _____

Course _____

Procedure 38 **Measuring a Rectal Temperature (Electronic Thermometer)**	Able to Perform	Able to Perform with Assistance	Unable to Perform	Initials and Date
1. Carry out beginning procedure actions. *Comments:*	☐	☐	☐	
2. Assemble equipment. *Comments:*	☐	☐	☐	
3. Lower the backrest of the bed. *Comments:*	☐	☐	☐	
4. Ask the patient to turn on his side, assisting if necessary. *Comments:*	☐	☐	☐	
5. Apply disposable gloves. *Comments:*	☐	☐	☐	
6. Place a small amount of lubricant on the tip of the sheath. *Comments:*	☐	☐	☐	
7. Fold the top bedclothes back to expose the patient's anal area. *Comments:*	☐	☐	☐	
8. Separate the buttocks with one hand. *Comments:*	☐	☐	☐	
9. Insert the sheath-covered probe gently 1 inch into the rectum and hold in place. *Comments:*	☐	☐	☐	
10. Replace the bedclothes for privacy. *Comments:*	☐	☐	☐	

continued on the following page

continued from the previous page

Procedure 38	Able to Perform	Able to Perform with Assistance	Unable to Perform	Initials and Date
11. Read the digital display when the buzzer signals that the temperature has been determined. *Comments:*	☐	☐	☐	
12. Remove the probe and discard the sheath. *Comments:*	☐	☐	☐	
13. Wipe lubricant from the patient and discard tissue. *Comments:*	☐	☐	☐	
14. Return the probe to its proper position. *Comments:*	☐	☐	☐	
15. Remove and discard gloves. *Comments:*	☐	☐	☐	
16. Record the temperature on a notepad. *Comments:*	☐	☐	☐	
17. Return the thermometer unit to the charger. *Comments:*	☐	☐	☐	
18. Carry out procedure completion actions. *Comments:*	☐	☐	☐	

Checklist for Procedure 39   Measuring an Axillary Temperature (Electronic Thermometer)

Name _____ Date _____

School _____

Instructor _____

Course _____

Procedure 39 Measuring an Axillary Temperature (Electronic Thermometer)	Able to Perform	Able to Perform with Assistance	Unable to Perform	Initials and Date
1. Carry out beginning procedure actions. Comments:	☐	☐	☐	
2. Assemble equipment. Comments:	☐	☐	☐	
3. Wipe the axillary area dry and put the covered probe in place. Comments:	☐	☐	☐	
4. Keep the patient's arm close to the body. Comments:	☐	☐	☐	
5. Hold the probe in place until the buzzer signals that the temperature has been recorded. Comments:	☐	☐	☐	
6. Remove the thermometer probe. Comments:	☐	☐	☐	
7. Dispose of the sheath. Comments:	☐	☐	☐	
8. Return the probe to its proper position. Comments:	☐	☐	☐	
9. Record the temperature on a notepad. Comments:	☐	☐	☐	
10. Return the thermometer unit to the charger. Comments:	☐	☐	☐	
11. Carry out procedure completion actions. Comments:	☐	☐	☐	

Checklist for Procedure 40   Measuring a Tympanic Temperature

Name _____ Date _____

School _____

Instructor _____

Course _____

Procedure 40 **Measuring a Tympanic Temperature**	Able to Perform	Able to Perform with Assistance	Unable to Perform	Initials and Date
1. Carry out beginning procedure actions. *Comments:*	☐	☐	☐	
2. Assemble equipment. *Comments:*	☐	☐	☐	
3. Place a clean probe cover on the probe. *Comments:*	☐	☐	☐	
4. Select the appropriate mode on the thermometer. *Comments:*	☐	☐	☐	
5. Check the lens to make sure it is clean and intact. *Comments:*	☐	☐	☐	
6. Apply gloves if contact with blood or body fluids is possible. *Comments:*	☐	☐	☐	
7. Position the patient so you have access to the ear you will be using. *Comments:*	☐	☐	☐	
8. Gently pull the ear pinna back and up. *Comments:*	☐	☐	☐	
9. Place the probe in the patient's ear, aiming it toward the tympanic membrane. *Comments:*	☐	☐	☐	
10. Insert the probe until it seals the ear canal. Do not apply pressure. *Comments:*	☐	☐	☐	

continued on the following page

continued from the previous page

Procedure 40	Able to Perform	Able to Perform with Assistance	Unable to Perform	Initials and Date
11. Rotate the probe handle slightly until it is aligned with the jaw. *Comments:*	☐	☐	☐	
12. Quickly press the activation button. *Comments:*	☐	☐	☐	
13. Leave the thermometer in the ear for the time recommended by the manufacturer. *Comments:*	☐	☐	☐	
14. When you have a reading, remove the probe and dispose of the cover. *Comments:*	☐	☐	☐	
15. Record the temperature on a notepad. *Comments:*	☐	☐	☐	
16. Return the thermometer unit to the charger. *Comments:*	☐	☐	☐	
17. Carry out procedure completion actions. *Comments:*	☐	☐	☐	

Checklist for Procedure 41 Cleaning Glass Thermometers

Name _____ Date _____

School _____

Instructor _____

Course _____

Procedure 41 Cleaning Glass Thermometers	Able to Perform	Able to Perform with Assistance	Unable to Perform	Initials and Date
1. Wash your hands. *Comments:*	☐	☐	☐	
2. Assemble equipment. *Comments:*	☐	☐	☐	
3. Take the tray of equipment to the soiled utility room. *Comments:*	☐	☐	☐	
4. Place a towel on the sink side. *Comments:*	☐	☐	☐	
5. Wash, dry and cover the container that is to be used for clean thermometers. *Comments:*	☐	☐	☐	
6. Place gauze in the bottom of the container. *Comments:*	☐	☐	☐	
7. Place a clean washbasin in the sink and line the bottom with a washcloth. *Comments:*	☐	☐	☐	
8. Fill the basin one-third full with cool water. *Comments:*	☐	☐	☐	
9. Apply disposable gloves. *Comments:*	☐	☐	☐	
10. Slowly turn on the cold water faucet. *Comments:*	☐	☐	☐	
11. Moisten a sponge/cotton ball and apply soap. *Comments:*	☐	☐	☐	

continued on the following page

continued from the previous page

Procedure 41	Able to Perform	Able to Perform with Assistance	Unable to Perform	Initials and Date
12. Pick up one thermometer at a time, holding it by the stem. *Comments:*	☐	☐	☐	
13. Using a circular motion, cleanse the thermometer from stem to bulb. *Comments:*	☐	☐	☐	
14. Discard cotton ball. *Comments:*	☐	☐	☐	
15. Carefully rinse the thermometer. *Comments:*	☐	☐	☐	
16. For each thermometer use a new, dry cotton ball for drying using a circular motion. *Comments:*	☐	☐	☐	
17. Check the thermometer for chips. *Comments:*	☐	☐	☐	
18. Shake each down to 96°F or below and place in the clean container. *Comments:*	☐	☐	☐	
19. Fill the container half full with disinfectant. *Comments:*	☐	☐	☐	
20. Empty the water from the dirty container. *Comments:*	☐	☐	☐	
21. Shut off the faucet. *Comments:*	☐	☐	☐	
22. Shut the basin drain and add hot water and soap. *Comments:*	☐	☐	☐	
23. Wash, rinse, and dry the dirty thermometer container and washbasin. *Comments:*	☐	☐	☐	
24. Remove gloves and discard. *Comments:*	☐	☐	☐	

Procedure 41	Able to Perform	Able to Perform with Assistance	Unable to Perform	Initials and Date
25. Add disinfectant so the each thermometer is completely covered by it. *Comments:*	☐	☐	☐	
26. Place a cover on the container. *Comments:*	☐	☐	☐	
27. Place a label with the date, time, and your initials on the container. *Comments:*	☐	☐	☐	
28. Place the towel in the laundry. *Comments:*	☐	☐	☐	
29. Dispose of used sponges or cotton balls in trash. *Comments:*	☐	☐	☐	
30. Leave the area neat and tidy. *Comments:*	☐	☐	☐	
31. After disinfecting, remove the label and thermometers. *Comments:*	☐	☐	☐	
32. Empty disinfectant. *Comments:*	☐	☐	☐	
33. Wash and dry the container. *Comments:*	☐	☐	☐	
34. Place a 4 × 4 folded sponge on the bottom of the container. *Comments:*	☐	☐	☐	
35. Rinse and dry the thermometers. *Comments:*	☐	☐	☐	
36. Place dry, clean thermometers on the sponge in the container and cover. *Comments:*	☐	☐	☐	
37. Store according to facility policy in clean area. *Comments:*	☐	☐	☐	
38. Wash your hands and report completion of task to the nurse. *Comments:*	☐	☐	☐	

Checklist for Procedure 42 Counting the Radial Pulse

Name _____ Date _____

School _____

Instructor _____

Course _____

Procedure 42 Counting the Radial Pulse	Able to Perform	Able to Perform with Assistance	Unable to Perform	Initials and Date
1. Carry out beginning procedure actions. *Comments:*	☐	☐	☐	
2. Place the patient in a comfortable position with the palm of the hand down and the arm resting on a flat surface. *Comments:*	☐	☐	☐	
3. With the tips of your first three fingers, locate the patient's pulse on the thumb side of the wrist. *Comments:*	☐	☐	☐	
4. When the pulse is felt, exert light pressure. Using the second hand of your watch, count for 1 minute. *Comments:*	☐	☐	☐	
5. Remember the reading when counting respirations. Document the reading as soon as possible. *Comments:*	☐	☐	☐	
6. Carry out procedure completion actions. *Comments:*	☐	☐	☐	

Checklist for Procedure 43 Counting the Apical-Radial Pulse

Name _____ Date _____

School _____

Instructor _____

Course _____

Procedure 43 Counting the Apical-Radial Pulse	Able to Perform	Able to Perform with Assistance	Unable to Perform	Initials and Date
1. Carry out beginning procedure actions. *Comments:*	☐	☐	☐	
2. Clean the stethoscope earpieces and bell with disinfectant. *Comments:*	☐	☐	☐	
3. Place the stethoscope earpieces in your ears with tips pointing slightly forward. *Comments:*	☐	☐	☐	
4. Place the stethoscope diaphragm or bell over the apex of the patient's heart. *Comments:*	☐	☐	☐	
5. Listen carefully for the heartbeat. *Comments:*	☐	☐	☐	
6. Count the louder sounding beats for 1 minute. *Comments:*	☐	☐	☐	
7. Check the radial pulse for 1 minute. *Comments:*	☐	☐	☐	
8. Document results on a notepad for comparison. *Comments:*	☐	☐	☐	
9. Clean the earpieces and bell of stethoscope with disinfectant. *Comments:*	☐	☐	☐	
10. Carry out procedure completion actions. *Comments:*	☐	☐	☐	

Checklist for Procedure 44   Counting Respirations

Name _____   Date _____

School _____

Instructor _____

Course _____

Procedure 44 Counting Respirations	Able to Perform	Able to Perform with Assistance	Unable to Perform	Initials and Date
1. When the pulse rate has been counted, leave your fingers on the radial pulse and start counting the number of times the chest rises and falls during 1 minute. *Comments:*	☐	☐	☐	
2. Note the depth and regularity of respirations. *Comments:*	☐	☐	☐	
3. Document the time, rate, depth, and regularity of respirations. *Comments:*	☐	☐	☐	

Checklist for Procedure 45   Taking Blood Pressure

Name _____ Date _____

School _____

Instructor _____

Course _____

Procedure 45 **Taking Blood Pressure**	Able to Perform	Able to Perform with Assistance	Unable to Perform	Initials and Date
1. Carry out beginning procedure actions. *Comments:*	☐	☐	☐	
2. Assemble equipment. *Comments:*	☐	☐	☐	
3. Remove the patient's arm from sleeve or roll sleeve 5 inches above the elbow. *Comments:*	☐	☐	☐	
4. Locate the brachial artery. *Comments:*	☐	☐	☐	
5. Place the patient's arm palm upward at heart level. *Comments:*	☐	☐	☐	
6. Wrap the cuff smoothly and snugly around the arm. *Comments:*	☐	☐	☐	
7. Center the bladder over the brachial artery 1 inch above the antecubital space. *Comments:*	☐	☐	☐	
8. Place the bulb in your dominant hand and feel for the radial pulse with the fingers of your other hand. *Comments:*	☐	☐	☐	
9. To find out how high to pump the cuff: Rapidly inflate the cuff until you no longer feel the radial pulse. Add 30 mm to that reading and note that point. *Comments:*	☐	☐	☐	
10. Quickly and steadily deflate the cuff and wait 15 to 30 seconds. *Comments:*	☐	☐	☐	
11. Place the stethoscope over the brachial artery. *Comments:*	☐	☐	☐	

continued on the following page

continued from the previous page

Procedure 45	Able to Perform	Able to Perform with Assistance	Unable to Perform	Initials and Date
12. Reinflate the cuff quickly and steadily to the level you calculated. *Comments:*	☐	☐	☐	
13. Release the air at an even pace. *Comments:*	☐	☐	☐	
14. Keep your eyes on the needle or the mercury. *Comments:*	☐	☐	☐	
15. Listen for the onset of at least two consecutive beats. *Comments:*	☐	☐	☐	
16. Note where the needle on the sphygmomanometer is when you hear the first sound. This is the systolic reading. *Comments:*	☐	☐	☐	
17. Continue deflating the cuff. *Comments:*	☐	☐	☐	
18. The last sound you hear is the diastolic reading. Continue to deflate and listen for 10 to 20 mm more to ensure correct reading. *Comments:*	☐	☐	☐	
19. Record the reading. *Comments:*	☐	☐	☐	
20. Wait 1 to 2 minutes if the procedure is to be repeated. *Comments:*	☐	☐	☐	
21. Clean the earpieces of the stethoscope with alcohol wipes, and if the tubing has contacted the patient or linen wipe it as well. *Comments:*	☐	☐	☐	
22. Return equipment to the appropriate area. *Comments:*	☐	☐	☐	
23. Carry out procedure completion actions. *Comments:*	☐	☐	☐	

Checklist for Procedure 46   Taking Blood Pressure with an Electronic Blood Pressure Apparatus

Name _____ Date _____

School _____

Instructor _____

Course _____

Procedure 46 **Taking Blood Pressure with an Electronic Blood Pressure Apparatus**	Able to Perform	Able to Perform with Assistance	Unable to Perform	Initials and Date
1. Carry out beginning procedure actions. *Comments:*	☐	☐	☐	
2. Assemble equipment. *Comments:*	☐	☐	☐	
3. Bring the electronic blood pressure unit to the patient's bedside and plug into a source of electricity. *Comments:*	☐	☐	☐	
4. Turn the machine on. *Comments:*	☐	☐	☐	
5. Select the appropriate cuff for the machine and size for the patient's extremity. *Comments:*	☐	☐	☐	
6. Remove restrictive clothing. *Comments:*	☐	☐	☐	
7. Squeeze excess air out of the cuff. *Comments:*	☐	☐	☐	
8. Connect the cuff to the connector hose. *Comments:*	☐	☐	☐	
9. Wrap the cuff snugly around the patient's extremity, making sure the "artery" arrow is correctly placed over the brachial artery. *Comments:*	☐	☐	☐	

continued on the following page

continued from the previous page

Procedure 46	Able to Perform	Able to Perform with Assistance	Unable to Perform	Initials and Date
10. Verify that the connector hose between the cuff and the machine is not kinked. *Comments:*	☐	☐	☐	
11. Set the frequency control for automatic or manual. *Comments:*	☐	☐	☐	
12. Press the start button. *Comments:*	☐	☐	☐	
13. If the cuff will take periodic, automatic measurements, set the designated frequency of blood pressure measurements. *Comments:*	☐	☐	☐	
14. Set the upper and lower alarm limits. *Comments:*	☐	☐	☐	
15. Remove the cuff at least every 2 hours and alternate sites, if possible. *Comments:*	☐	☐	☐	
16. Evaluate the skin for redness and irritation. *Comments:*	☐	☐	☐	
17. Report abnormalities to the nurse. *Comments:*	☐	☐	☐	
18. Carry out procedure completion actions. *Comments:*	☐	☐	☐	

Checklist for Procedure 47   Weighing and Measuring the Patient using an Upright Scale

Name _____ Date _____

School _____

Instructor _____

Course _____

Procedure 47 Weighing and Measuring the Patient using an Upright Scale	Able to Perform	Able to Perform with Assistance	Unable to Perform	Initials and Date
1. Carry out beginning procedure actions. *Comments:*	☐	☐	☐	
2. Check notes or chart for previous weight as documented. *Comments:*	☐	☐	☐	
3. Escort the patient to the scales. *Comments:*	☐	☐	☐	
4. Place a paper towel on the platform of the scale. *Comments:*	☐	☐	☐	
5. Check to be sure the weights are to the extreme left and the balance bar is hanging free. *Comments:*	☐	☐	☐	
6. Assist the patient with removing shoes and step up onto the scale platform. *Comments:*	☐	☐	☐	
7. Instruct the patient not to hold onto any part of the scale. *Comments:*	☐	☐	☐	
8. Move the large weight to the right to the closest estimated patient weight. *Comments:*	☐	☐	☐	
9. Move the small weight to the right until the balance bar hangs freely halfway between the upper and lower guides. *Comments:*	☐	☐	☐	

continued on the following page

continued from the previous page

Procedure 47	Able to Perform	Able to Perform with Assistance	Unable to Perform	Initials and Date
10. Add the two figures and record the weight. *Comments:*	☐	☐	☐	
11. Assist the patient with turning on the platform until facing away from the balance bar. *Comments:*	☐	☐	☐	
12. Raise the height bar until it is level with the top of the patient's head. *Comments:*	☐	☐	☐	
13. Read the height at the movable point of the ruler. *Comments:*	☐	☐	☐	
14. Note the number of inches indicated and record on your notepad. *Comments:*	☐	☐	☐	
15. Assist the patient off the platform. *Comments:*	☐	☐	☐	
16. Help the patient to put on shoes and return to room. *Comments:*	☐	☐	☐	
17. Carry out procedure completion actions. *Comments:*	☐	☐	☐	

Checklist for Procedure 48 Weighing the Patient on a Chair Scale

Name _____ Date _____

School _____

Instructor _____

Course _____

Procedure 48 Weighing the Patient on a Chair Scale	Able to Perform	Able to Perform with Assistance	Unable to Perform	Initials and Date
1. Carry out beginning procedure actions. *Comments:*	☐	☐	☐	
2. Assemble equipment. *Comments:*	☐	☐	☐	
3. Take the patient in a wheelchair to the chair scale. *Comments:*	☐	☐	☐	
4. Lock the wheelchair brakes. *Comments:*	☐	☐	☐	
5. Check the chair scale brakes to make sure they are locked. *Comments:*	☐	☐	☐	
6. Apply a transfer belt to the patient. *Comments:*	☐	☐	☐	
7. Assist in a pivot transfer to the chair on the scale. *Comments:*	☐	☐	☐	
8. Instruct the patient to sit down when the chair is felt against the back of the legs. *Comments:*	☐	☐	☐	
9. Check to ensure the patient's feet are on the footrest of the scale. *Comments:*	☐	☐	☐	
10. Walk behind the scale to obtain the reading. *Comments:*	☐	☐	☐	
11. Transfer the patient back to the wheelchair. *Comments:*	☐	☐	☐	
12. Carry out procedure completion actions. *Comments:*	☐	☐	☐	

Checklist for Procedure 49 Measuring Weight with an Electronic Wheelchair Scale

Name _____ Date _____

School _____

Instructor _____

Course _____

Procedure 49 **Measuring Weight with an Electronic Wheelchair Scale**	Able to Perform	Able to Perform with Assistance	Unable to Perform	Initials and Date
1. Carry out beginning procedure actions. *Comments:*	☐	☐	☐	
2. Assemble equipment. *Comments:*	☐	☐	☐	
3. Determine the empty weight of a wheelchair by weighing it on the scale. *Comments:*	☐	☐	☐	
4. Take the wheelchair to the patient's room. *Comments:*	☐	☐	☐	
5. Help the patient into the wheelchair and take her to the electronic wheelchair scale. *Comments:*	☐	☐	☐	
6. Open the metal ramp sides on the scale to rest on the floor. *Comments:*	☐	☐	☐	
7. Press the "on" button. *Comments:*	☐	☐	☐	
8. Roll the patient onto the platform of the scale. *Comments:*	☐	☐	☐	
9. Lock wheelchair wheels. *Comments:*	☐	☐	☐	
10. The digital readout will show the weight. *Comments:*	☐	☐	☐	

continued on the following page

continued from the previous page

Procedure 49	Able to Perform	Able to Perform with Assistance	Unable to Perform	Initials and Date
11. Record the weight of the patient in the wheelchair. *Comments:*	☐	☐	☐	
12. Subtract the empty wheelchair weight to obtain the patient's weight. *Comments:*	☐	☐	☐	
13. Unlock the wheelchair wheels. *Comments:*	☐	☐	☐	
14. Roll the wheelchair with the patient off the scale. *Comments:*	☐	☐	☐	
15. Fold the scale ramps back into place. *Comments:*	☐	☐	☐	
16. Carry out procedure completion actions. *Comments:*	☐	☐	☐	

Checklist for Procedure 50　Measuring and Weighing the Patient in Bed

Name _____ Date _____

School _____

Instructor _____

Course _____

Procedure 50 Measuring and Weighing the Patient in Bed	Able to Perform	Able to Perform with Assistance	Unable to Perform	Initials and Date
1. Carry out beginning procedure actions. *Comments:*	☐	☐	☐	
2. Obtain assistance from a coworker. *Comments:*	☐	☐	☐	
3. Assemble equipment. *Comments:*	☐	☐	☐	
4. Check scale sling and straps for frayed areas or straps that do not close properly. *Comments:*	☐	☐	☐	
5. Lower the side rail on your side. *Comments:*	☐	☐	☐	
6. Check that the opposite side rail is up. *Comments:*	☐	☐	☐	
7. Fanfold top linen to the foot of the bed. *Comments:*	☐	☐	☐	
8. Position the patient flat on his back with arms and legs straight and body in good alignment. *Comments:*	☐	☐	☐	
9. Make a small pencil mark at the top of the patient's head on the sheet. *Comments:*	☐	☐	☐	
10. Make a second pencil mark even with the heels. *Comments:*	☐	☐	☐	
11. Roll the patient on his side. *Comments:*	☐	☐	☐	

continued on the following page

continued from the previous page

Procedure 50	Able to Perform	Able to Perform with Assistance	Unable to Perform	Initials and Date
12. Use a tape measure to measure the distance between the two marks. *Comments:*	☐	☐	☐	
13. Note the patient's height in feet and inches on a notepad. *Comments:*	☐	☐	☐	
14. Cover the canvas sling with a sheet. *Comments:*	☐	☐	☐	
15. Balance the scale. *Comments:*	☐	☐	☐	
16. Remove the scale sling and position half of the sheet-covered sling under the patient. *Comments:*	☐	☐	☐	
17. Turn the patient away from you. *Comments:*	☐	☐	☐	
18. Place the sling under the patient. *Comments:*	☐	☐	☐	
19. Return the patient to recumbent position and place the sling so the patient rests securely within it. *Comments:*	☐	☐	☐	
20. Attach the sling to the suspension straps and check for security. *Comments:*	☐	☐	☐	
21. Position the lift frame over the bed with the base legs in maximum position. *Comments:*	☐	☐	☐	
22. Lock the frame. *Comments:*	☐	☐	☐	
23. Elevate the head of the bed and bring the patient to a sitting position. *Comments:*	☐	☐	☐	

Procedure 50	Able to Perform	Able to Perform with Assistance	Unable to Perform	Initials and Date
24. Attach the suspension straps to the frame. *Comments:*	☐	☐	☐	
25. Position the patient's arms inside the straps. *Comments:*	☐	☐	☐	
26. Slowly raise the sling so the patient's body is off the bed. *Comments:*	☐	☐	☐	
27. Guide the lift away from the bed so that no part of the patient touches the bed. *Comments:*	☐	☐	☐	
28. Take and note the reading. *Comments:*	☐	☐	☐	
29. Reposition the sling over the center of the bed. *Comments:*	☐	☐	☐	
30. Release the knob slowly, lowering the patient to the bed. *Comments:*	☐	☐	☐	
31. Remove the sling by reversing the process in steps 16–20. *Comments:*	☐	☐	☐	
32. Assist the patient to a comfortable position. *Comments:*	☐	☐	☐	
33. Move the overbed scale out of the way. *Comments:*	☐	☐	☐	
34. Replace the top bed linen over the patient. *Comments:*	☐	☐	☐	
35. Raise the side rail and lower the bed to the lowest horizontal height. *Comments:*	☐	☐	☐	
36. Carry out procedure completion actions. *Comments:*	☐	☐	☐	

Checklist for Procedure 51   Admitting the Patient

Name _____ Date _____

School _____

Instructor _____

Course _____

Procedure 51 **Admitting the Patient**	Able to Perform	Able to Perform with Assistance	Unable to Perform	Initials and Date
1. Wash hands. *Comments:*	☐	☐	☐	
2. Assemble equipment. *Comments:*	☐	☐	☐	
3. Make sure that all necessary equipment and furniture are in the unit. *Comments:*	☐	☐	☐	
4. Check that the equipment and furniture are in their proper places and in good working order. *Comments:*	☐	☐	☐	
5. Check the unit for adequate lighting. *Comments:*	☐	☐	☐	
6. Loosen the top linen at the foot of the bed. *Comments:*	☐	☐	☐	
7. Open the bed. *Comments:*	☐	☐	☐	
8. Identify the patient and introduce yourself. *Comments:*	☐	☐	☐	
9. Take the patient and the patient's family to the unit. *Comments:*	☐	☐	☐	
10. Do not rush the patient. *Comments:*	☐	☐	☐	

continued on the following page

continued from the previous page

Procedure 51	Able to Perform	Able to Perform with Assistance	Unable to Perform	Initials and Date
11. Be courteous and helpful to the patient and the family. *Comments:*	☐	☐	☐	
12. If the patient is ambulatory, offer a chair. *Comments:*	☐	☐	☐	
13. Ask the family to wait in the lounge or lobby during patient admission. *Comments:*	☐	☐	☐	
14. Unless the room is private, introduce the patient to the other patients in the room. *Comments:*	☐	☐	☐	
15. As permitted, explain what will happen in the next hour. *Comments:*	☐	☐	☐	
16. Screen the unit to provide privacy. *Comments:*	☐	☐	☐	
17. Help the patient to undress and put on a hospital gown. Care for clothing according to facility policy. *Comments:*	☐	☐	☐	
18. Check the patient's vital signs, weight, and height. *Comments:*	☐	☐	☐	
19. Assist the patient into bed. *Comments:*	☐	☐	☐	
20. Adjust the side rails as needed. *Comments:*	☐	☐	☐	
21. If the patient is wearing any jewelry or has valuables, make a list of them and ask the patient sign it. *Comments:*	☐	☐	☐	
22. Ask the relatives to sign the list also and either take valuables home or place them in the hospital safe. *Comments:*	☐	☐	☐	

Procedure 51	Able to Perform	Able to Perform with Assistance	Unable to Perform	Initials and Date
23. If a urine specimen is necessary, put on gloves and assist the patient as necessary. Allow the patient to use the bathroom or offer the bedpan or urinal. *Comments:*	☐	☐	☐	
24. If the bedpan is used, pour the patient's specimen from the bedpan into the specimen bottle and put on the cap. *Comments:*	☐	☐	☐	
25. Remove and dispose of gloves. *Comments:*	☐	☐	☐	
26. Label the specimen correctly. *Comments:*	☐	☐	☐	
27. Complete an admission form. *Comments:*	☐	☐	☐	
28. If the patient is being admitted to a long-term care facility, label clothing and complete the personal belongings inventory form. *Comments:*	☐	☐	☐	
29. Orient the patient to the unit. *Comments:*	☐	☐	☐	
30. Carry out procedure completion actions. *Comments:*	☐	☐	☐	

Checklist for Procedure 52   Transferring the Patient

Name _____   Date _____

School _____

Instructor _____

Course _____

Procedure 52 Transferring the Patient	Able to Perform	Able to Perform with Assistance	Unable to Perform	Initials and Date
1. Find out which unit the patient is transferring to and check to see that it is ready. *Comments:*	☐	☐	☐	
2. Check to see the method of transport and get the necessary vehicle. *Comments:*	☐	☐	☐	
3. Check to see if any equipment is to be transferred with the patient. *Comments:*	☐	☐	☐	
4. Carry out beginning procedure actions. *Comments:*	☐	☐	☐	
5. Explain to the patient what you are doing. *Comments:*	☐	☐	☐	
6. Gather all the patient's belongings and check against the clothes list. Place disposables in a paper bag. *Comments:*	☐	☐	☐	
7. Assist the patient with putting on a robe and slippers. *Comments:*	☐	☐	☐	
8. Assist the patient into a wheelchair or stretcher. *Comments:*	☐	☐	☐	
9. If the entire bed is used, make sure the side rails are up. *Comments:*	☐	☐	☐	
10. Obtain the patient's chart, nursing care plan, medications, and paper bag from the nurse. *Comments:*	☐	☐	☐	

continued on the following page

continued from the previous page

Procedure 52	Able to Perform	Able to Perform with Assistance	Unable to Perform	Initials and Date
11. Transport the patient and her belongings to the new unit. *Comments:*	☐	☐	☐	
12. Give the patient's chart, nursing care plan, and medications to the nurse in charge. *Comments:*	☐	☐	☐	
13. Introduce the patient to the staff. *Comments:*	☐	☐	☐	
14. Proceed to the patient's room. *Comments:*	☐	☐	☐	
15. Assist staff in helping the patient into bed, putting away the patient's belongings, and getting the patient settled. *Comments:*	☐	☐	☐	
16. Carry out procedure completion actions. *Comments:*	☐	☐	☐	

Checklist for Procedure 53   Discharging the Patient

Name _____ Date _____

School _____

Instructor _____

Course _____

Procedure 53 **Discharging the Patient**	Able to Perform	Able to Perform with Assistance	Unable to Perform	Initials and Date
1. Check to see if a discharge order has been written. *Comments:*	☐	☐	☐	
2. Carry out beginning procedure actions. *Comments:*	☐	☐	☐	
3. Assemble equipment. *Comments:*	☐	☐	☐	
4. Help the patient to dress, if necessary. *Comments:*	☐	☐	☐	
5. Collect the patient's personal belongings and check them against the admission list. *Comments:*	☐	☐	☐	
6. Pack, if necessary. *Comments:*	☐	☐	☐	
7. Check valuables against the admission list. *Comments:*	☐	☐	☐	
8. Make sure all belongings are out of the closet and drawers. *Comments:*	☐	☐	☐	
9. Check to see if medications or equipment are to be sent home with the patient. *Comments:*	☐	☐	☐	
10. Verify that the patient has received discharge instructions. *Comments:*	☐	☐	☐	

continued on the following page

continued from the previous page

Procedure 53	Able to Perform	Able to Perform with Assistance	Unable to Perform	Initials and Date
11. If valuables are in the facility safe, instruct the patient or family member on how to collect them. *Comments:*	☐	☐	☐	
12. Help the patient into a wheelchair. *Comments:*	☐	☐	☐	
13. Take the patient to the discharge entrance of the facility. *Comments:*	☐	☐	☐	
14. Help the patient to transfer safely into the vehicle. *Comments:*	☐	☐	☐	
15. Be gracious as you say goodbye. *Comments:*	☐	☐	☐	
16. Return the wheelchair. *Comments:*	☐	☐	☐	
17. Return to the patient unit. *Comments:*	☐	☐	☐	
18. Strip the bed and dispose of the linen. *Comments:*	☐	☐	☐	
19. Clean and replace equipment used in patient care. *Comments:*	☐	☐	☐	
20. Wash your hands. *Comments:*	☐	☐	☐	
21. Record the discharge. *Comments:*	☐	☐	☐	
22. Report completion of the task to the nurse. *Comments:*	☐	☐	☐	

Checklist for Procedure 54   Making a Closed Bed

Name _____ Date _____

School _____

Instructor _____

Course _____

Procedure 54 Making a Closed Bed	Able to Perform	Able to Perform with Assistance	Unable to Perform	Initials and Date
1. Wash your hands and assemble equipment. *Comments:*	☐	☐	☐	
2. Elevate the bed to a comfortable working height and lock bed wheels. *Comments:*	☐	☐	☐	
3. Arrange linen on a chair at the bedside in the order in which it is to be used. *Comments:*	☐	☐	☐	
4. Position the mattress to the head of the bed. *Comments:*	☐	☐	☐	
5. Place a mattress cover on the mattress, if used. *Comments:*	☐	☐	☐	
6. Place the mattress pad even with the top of the mattress and unfold it. *Comments:*	☐	☐	☐	
7. Place the bottom sheet on the bed and unfold it, seam side down, and wide hem at the top. *Comments:*	☐	☐	☐	
8. Tuck 12 to 18 inches of the sheet smoothly over the top of the mattress. *Comments:*	☐	☐	☐	
9. Make a mitered corner. *Comments:*	☐	☐	☐	

continued on the following page

continued from the previous page

Procedure 54	Able to Perform	Able to Perform with Assistance	Unable to Perform	Initials and Date
10. Tuck in the sheet on one side, keeping the sheet straight and working from the head to the foot of the bed. *Comments:*	☐	☐	☐	
11. If used, place a plastic draw sheet and half sheet with the upper edge 14 inches under the head of the mattress and tuck under one side. *Comments:*	☐	☐	☐	
12. Unfold and place the top sheet on the bed, seam up, top hem even with the upper edge of the mattress and center fold in the center of the bed. *Comments:*	☐	☐	☐	
13. Spread the blanket over the top sheet and foot mattress. *Comments:*	☐	☐	☐	
14. Tuck the top sheet and blanket under the mattress at the foot of the bed, making a square corner. *Comments:*	☐	☐	☐	
15. Place the spread with its top hem even with the head of the mattress. Unfold the spread to the foot of the bed. *Comments:*	☐	☐	☐	
16. Tuck the spread under the mattress at the foot of the bed and miter the corner. *Comments:*	☐	☐	☐	
17. Go to the other side of the bed. Fanfold the top covers to the center of the bed so you can work with the lower sheets and pad. *Comments:*	☐	☐	☐	
18. Tuck the bottom sheet under the head of the mattress and miter the corner. *Comments:*	☐	☐	☐	
19. Tuck the protective draw sheet and cotton draw sheet under the mattress. *Comments:*	☐	☐	☐	

Procedure 54	Able to Perform	Able to Perform with Assistance	Unable to Perform	Initials and Date
20. Tuck in the top sheet and blanket at the foot of the bed and miter the corner. *Comments:*	☐	☐	☐	
21. Fold the top sheet back over the blanket, making an 8-inch cuff. *Comments:*	☐	☐	☐	
22. Tuck in the spread at the foot of the bed and miter the corner. Bring the top of the spread to the head of the mattress. *Comments:*	☐	☐	☐	
23. Insert the pillow in the pillowcase. *Comments:*	☐	☐	☐	
24. Place the pillow at the head of the bed with the open end away from the door. *Comments:*	☐	☐	☐	
25. Lower the bed to its lowest position. *Comments:*	☐	☐	☐	
26. Arrange the room, leaving it neat and tidy. *Comments:*	☐	☐	☐	
27. Wash your hands. *Comments:*	☐	☐	☐	
28. Report the completion of your task to your supervisor. *Comments:*	☐	☐	☐	

Checklist for Procedure 55   Opening the Closed Bed

Name _____ Date _____

School _____

Instructor _____

Course _____

Procedure 55 **Opening the Closed Bed**	Able to Perform	Able to Perform with Assistance	Unable to Perform	Initials and Date
1. Wash your hands. *Comments:*	☐	☐	☐	
2. Check assignment for bed location. *Comments:*	☐	☐	☐	
3. Raise the bed to a comfortable working height. Lock the wheels. *Comments:*	☐	☐	☐	
4. Loosen the top bedding. *Comments:*	☐	☐	☐	
5. Facing the head of the bed, grasp the top sheet and spread and fanfold it to the foot of the bed. *Comments:*	☐	☐	☐	
6. Return the bed to the lowest horizontal position. *Comments:*	☐	☐	☐	
7. Place the overbed table over the foot of the bed. *Comments:*	☐	☐	☐	
8. Place the call bell near the pillow or within easy reach. *Comments:*	☐	☐	☐	
9. Leave the unit neat and tidy. *Comments:*	☐	☐	☐	
10. Wash your hands. *Comments:*	☐	☐	☐	
11. Report completion of the task to your supervisor. *Comments:*	☐	☐	☐	

Checklist for Procedure 56   Making an Occupied Bed

Name _____ Date _____

School _____

Instructor _____

Course _____

Procedure 56 Making an Occupied Bed	Able to Perform	Able to Perform with Assistance	Unable to Perform	Initials and Date
1. Carry out beginning procedure actions. *Comments:*	☐	☐	☐	
2. Assemble your equipment. *Comments:*	☐	☐	☐	
3. Place the bedside chair at the foot of the bed. *Comments:*	☐	☐	☐	
4. Arrange clean linen on the chair in the order in which it is to be used. *Comments:*	☐	☐	☐	
5. Raise the bed to a comfortable working height. *Comments:*	☐	☐	☐	
6. Lower the side rail. *Comments:*	☐	☐	☐	
7. Loosen the bedclothes on your side. *Comments:*	☐	☐	☐	
8. Put the side rail up and go to the opposite side of the bed. *Comments:*	☐	☐	☐	
9. Adjust the mattress to the head of the bed. *Comments:*	☐	☐	☐	
10. Remove the top covers except for the top sheet one at a time. *Comments:*	☐	☐	☐	
11. Place a clean sheet or bath blanket over the top sheet. *Comments:*	☐	☐	☐	
12. Slide the soiled sheet out, from top to bottom. *Comments:*	☐	☐	☐	

continued on the following page

continued from the previous page

Procedure 56	Able to Perform	Able to Perform with Assistance	Unable to Perform	Initials and Date
13. Ask the patient to move to the side of the bed toward you. *Comments:*	☐	☐	☐	
14. Go to the other side of the bed. *Comments:*	☐	☐	☐	
15. Fanfold the soiled cotton draw sheet and bottom sheet close to the patient. *Comments:*	☐	☐	☐	
16. Straighten the mattress pad. *Comments:*	☐	☐	☐	
17. Place a clean sheet on the bed so that the narrow hem comes to the edge of the mattress at the foot with the seamed side of the hem toward the bed and the lengthwise center fold of the sheet at the center of the bed. *Comments:*	☐	☐	☐	
18. Fanfold the opposite side of the sheet close to the patient. *Comments:*	☐	☐	☐	
19. Tuck the top of the sheet under the head of the mattress. *Comments:*	☐	☐	☐	
20. Make a mitered corner. *Comments:*	☐	☐	☐	
21. Tuck the side of the sheet under the mattress, working toward the foot of the bed. *Comments:*	☐	☐	☐	
22. Position a fresh draw sheet. Tuck it under the mattress. *Comments:*	☐	☐	☐	
23. Ask or assist the patient to roll toward you, over the fanfolded linen. *Comments:*	☐	☐	☐	
24. Raise the side rails. *Comments:*	☐	☐	☐	
25. Go to the other side of the bed. Lower the side rail. *Comments:*	☐	☐	☐	

Procedure 56	Able to Perform	Able to Perform with Assistance	Unable to Perform	Initials and Date
26. Remove the soiled linen by rolling the edges inward. *Comments:*	☐	☐	☐	
27. Remove gloves and discard according to facility policy. *Comments:*	☐	☐	☐	
28. Wash your hands. *Comments:*	☐	☐	☐	
29. Pull the clean bottom sheet into place. Tuck it under the mattress and make a mitered corner. *Comments:*	☐	☐	☐	
30. Pull gently to eliminate wrinkles; then tuck the side of the sheet under the mattress, working from top to bottom. *Comments:*	☐	☐	☐	
31. Pull the draw sheet smoothly into place, tucking it firmly under the mattress. *Comments:*	☐	☐	☐	
32. Place the top sheet over the patient. *Comments:*	☐	☐	☐	
33. Remove the bath blanket. *Comments:*	☐	☐	☐	
34. Complete the bed as an unoccupied bed. *Comments:*	☐	☐	☐	
35. Assist the patient to turn on her back. *Comments:*	☐	☐	☐	
36. Place a clean pillowcase on the pillow that is not being used. Replace that pillow. *Comments:*	☐	☐	☐	
37. Change the other pillowcase. *Comments:*	☐	☐	☐	
38. Carry out procedure completion actions. *Comments:*	☐	☐	☐	

Checklist for Procedure 57   Making the Surgical Bed

Name _____ Date _____

School _____

Instructor _____

Course _____

Procedure 57 Making the Surgical Bed	Able to Perform	Able to Perform with Assistance	Unable to Perform	Initials and Date
1. Wash your hands. *Comments:*	☐	☐	☐	
2. Check assignment for unit location. *Comments:*	☐	☐	☐	
3. Assemble your equipment. *Comments:*	☐	☐	☐	
4. Lock the bed. *Comments:*	☐	☐	☐	
5. Apply gloves if linen is wet or soiled with blood or body fluids. *Comments:*	☐	☐	☐	
6. Strip and discard used linen. *Comments:*	☐	☐	☐	
7. Remove gloves and discard according to facility policy. *Comments:*	☐	☐	☐	
8. Wash your hands. *Comments:*	☐	☐	☐	
9. Make the bottom foundation bed. Repeat on the opposite side of the bed. *Comments:*	☐	☐	☐	
10. Place a protective draw sheet over the head of the mattress sheet. Cover with a cotton draw sheet. Miter the corners and tuck sheets in on the sides. *Comments:*	☐	☐	☐	

continued on the following page

continued from the previous page

Procedure 57	Able to Perform	Able to Perform with Assistance	Unable to Perform	Initials and Date
11. Place the top sheet, blanket, and spread in the usual manner. Do not tuck them in. *Comments:*	☐	☐	☐	
12. Fold the linen back at the foot of the bed even with the edge of the mattress. *Comments:*	☐	☐	☐	
13. Fanfold the upper covers and top sheet to the far side of the bed. *Comments:*	☐	☐	☐	
14. Tie a waterproof pillow to the head of the bed with gauze bandaging or place according to facility policy. *Comments:*	☐	☐	☐	
15. Arrange the room so that you may position a stretcher next to the bed. *Comments:*	☐	☐	☐	
16. Leave the bed locked and at the same height as the stretcher. *Comments:*	☐	☐	☐	
17. Check the unit for obvious hazards. *Comments:*	☐	☐	☐	
18. Leave the room neat and tidy. *Comments:*	☐	☐	☐	
19. Wash your hands. *Comments:*	☐	☐	☐	
20. Report completion of the task to your supervisor. *Comments:*	☐	☐	☐	

Checklist for Procedure 58   Assisting with the Tub Bath or Shower

Name _____ Date _____

School _____

Instructor _____

Course _____

Procedure 58 Assisting with the Tub Bath or Shower	Able to Perform	Able to Perform with Assistance	Unable to Perform	Initials and Date
1. Carry out beginning procedure actions. *Comments:*	☐	☐	☐	
2. Assemble necessary equipment and supplies and take them to the bathroom. *Comments:*	☐	☐	☐	
3. Prepare the bathtub, making sure it is clean. *Comments:*	☐	☐	☐	
4. Fill the tub half full of water or adjust the shower flow. *Comments:*	☐	☐	☐	
5. Check the water temperature with a thermometer or your wrist or elbow. The water should feel comfortably warm or approximately 105°F. *Comments:*	☐	☐	☐	
6. Help the patient put on a robe and slippers. Cover the nonambulatory patient with a bath blanket. *Comments:*	☐	☐	☐	
7. Escort the patient to the bathroom. *Comments:*	☐	☐	☐	
8. Help the patient to undress. *Comments:*	☐	☐	☐	
9. Give the patient a towel to wrap around the waist. *Comments:*	☐	☐	☐	
10. Position a shower chair in the tub or shower, if needed. *Comments:*	☐	☐	☐	
11. Assist the patient into the tub or shower. *Comments:*	☐	☐	☐	

continued on the following page

continued from the previous page

Procedure 58	Able to Perform	Able to Perform with Assistance	Unable to Perform	Initials and Date
12. If the patient has open skin lesions, apply gloves. *Comments:*	☐	☐	☐	
13. Encourage the patient to wash his body. Assist as needed. *Comments:*	☐	☐	☐	
14. Wash the patient's back, observing the skin for signs of redness or breaks. *Comments:*	☐	☐	☐	
15. Allow the patient to wash the genitalia, if able. If the patient is unable, apply gloves, wash the genitalia, remove gloves, then wash hands. *Comments:*	☐	☐	☐	
16. Shampoo the patient's hair if the patient wishes and you have permission to do so. *Comments:*	☐	☐	☐	
17. Hold the bath blanket around the patient as he steps from the tub. *Comments:*	☐	☐	☐	
18. Assist the patient to dry, apply deodorant, dress, and return to the unit. *Comments:*	☐	☐	☐	
19. Escort the patient back to his unit. *Comments:*	☐	☐	☐	
20. Return supplies to the patient's unit. *Comments:*	☐	☐	☐	
21. Carry out procedure completion actions. *Comments:*	☐	☐	☐	
22. Apply gloves to clean and disinfect the tub or shower. *Comments:*	☐	☐	☐	
23. Discard soiled linen. *Comments:*	☐	☐	☐	
24. Wash your hands. *Comments:*	☐	☐	☐	

continued from the previous page

Checklist for Procedure 59   Bed Bath

Name _____ Date _____

School _____

Instructor _____

Course _____

Procedure 59 Bed Bath	Able to Perform	Able to Perform with Assistance	Unable to Perform	Initials and Date
1. Carry out beginning procedure actions. *Comments:*	☐	☐	☐	
2. Assemble your equipment. *Comments:*	☐	☐	☐	
3. Close the windows and door to prevent chilling. *Comments:*	☐	☐	☐	
4. Close the privacy curtain. *Comments:*	☐	☐	☐	
5. Place clean towels and linen on a chair in the order of use. *Comments:*	☐	☐	☐	
6. Place a laundry hamper nearby. *Comments:*	☐	☐	☐	
7. Offer the bedpan or urinal. *Comments:*	☐	☐	☐	
8. Lower the head of the bed and the side rail on the side where you are working. *Comments:*	☐	☐	☐	
9. Loosen the top bedclothes. *Comments:*	☐	☐	☐	
10. Remove and fold the blanket and spread and place them over the back of the chair. *Comments:*	☐	☐	☐	

continued on the following page

continued from the previous page

Procedure 59	Able to Perform	Able to Perform with Assistance	Unable to Perform	Initials and Date
11. Leave one pillow under the patient's head. Place the other on a chair. *Comments:*	☐	☐	☐	
12. Remove the patient's nightwear and place it in a laundry hamper. *Comments:*	☐	☐	☐	
13. Fill a bath basin two-thirds full of water at 105°F. *Comments:*	☐	☐	☐	
14. Assist the patient to move to the side of the bed nearest you. *Comments:*	☐	☐	☐	
15. Fold a face towel over the upper edge of the bath blanket to keep the blanket dry. *Comments:*	☐	☐	☐	
16. Apply disposable gloves. *Comments:*	☐	☐	☐	
17. Form a mitt by folding a washcloth around your hand. *Comments:*	☐	☐	☐	
18. Wet the washcloth. *Comments:*	☐	☐	☐	
19. Wash around the eyes, using separate corners of the cloth for each eye. *Comments:*	☐	☐	☐	
20. Rinse the washcloth and apply soap if the patient desires. *Comments:*	☐	☐	☐	
21. Wash and rinse the patient's face, ears, and neck. Use a towel to dry. *Comments:*	☐	☐	☐	

Procedure 59	Able to Perform	Able to Perform with Assistance	Unable to Perform	Initials and Date
22. Remove gloves and discard according to facility policy. *Comments:*	☐	☐	☐	
23. Expose the patient's far arm. *Comments:*	☐	☐	☐	
24. Place a bath towel underneath the arm. *Comments:*	☐	☐	☐	
25. Wash, rinse, and pat dry the arm and hand. *Comments:*	☐	☐	☐	
26. Make sure the axilla is clean and dry. *Comments:*	☐	☐	☐	
27. Repeat for other arm. *Comments:*	☐	☐	☐	
28. Apply deodorant if the patient requests it. *Comments:*	☐	☐	☐	
29. Care for hands and nails as necessary. *Comments:*	☐	☐	☐	
30. Discard used bath water and refill the basin two-thirds full with water at 105°F. *Comments:*	☐	☐	☐	
31. Place a bath towel over the patient's chest; then fold the blanket to the waist. *Comments:*	☐	☐	☐	
32. Under the towel, wash, rinse, and pat dry the chest. *Comments:*	☐	☐	☐	
33. Fold the bath blanket down to the pubic area. *Comments:*	☐	☐	☐	

continued on the following page

continued from the previous page

Procedure 59	Able to Perform	Able to Perform with Assistance	Unable to Perform	Initials and Date
34. Wash, rinse, and pat dry the abdomen. *Comments:*	☐	☐	☐	
35. Fold the bath blanket up to cover the abdomen and chest. *Comments:*	☐	☐	☐	
36. Slide the towel out from under the bath blanket. *Comments:*	☐	☐	☐	
37. Ask the patient to flex the far knee, if possible. *Comments:*	☐	☐	☐	
38. Fold the bath blanket up to expose the thigh, leg, and foot. *Comments:*	☐	☐	☐	
39. Protect the bed with a bath towel. *Comments:*	☐	☐	☐	
40. Place the bath basin on the towel. *Comments:*	☐	☐	☐	
41. Place the patient's foot in the basin. *Comments:*	☐	☐	☐	
42. Wash and rinse the leg and foot. *Comments:*	☐	☐	☐	
43. Lift the leg and move the basin to the other side of the bed. *Comments:*	☐	☐	☐	
44. Dry the leg and foot, drying well between toes. *Comments:*	☐	☐	☐	
45. Repeat for the other leg and foot. *Comments:*	☐	☐	☐	
46. Remove the basin from the bed before drying the leg and foot. *Comments:*	☐	☐	☐	

Procedure 59	Able to Perform	Able to Perform with Assistance	Unable to Perform	Initials and Date
47. Care for toenails as necessary. *Comments:*	☐	☐	☐	
48. Change water and check for correct temperature. *Comments:*	☐	☐	☐	
49. Help the patient to turn on the side away from you, toward the center of the bed. *Comments:*	☐	☐	☐	
50. Place a bath towel lengthwise next to the patient's back and wash, rinse, and dry neck, back, and buttocks. *Comments:*	☐	☐	☐	
51. A backrub is usually given at this time. *Comments:*	☐	☐	☐	
52. Help the patient to turn on the back. *Comments:*	☐	☐	☐	
53. Place a towel under the buttocks and upper legs. *Comments:*	☐	☐	☐	
54. Change the water in the basin and check for correct temperature. *Comments:*	☐	☐	☐	
55. Place a washcloth, soap, basin, and bath towel within reach of the patient so she can wash the genitalia. Assist the patient as necessary. *Comments:*	☐	☐	☐	
56. Remove gloves and discard according to facility policy. *Comments:*	☐	☐	☐	
57. Carry out range of motion exercises. *Comments:*	☐	☐	☐	
58. Cover the pillow with a towel. *Comments:*	☐	☐	☐	

continued on the following page

continued from the previous page

Procedure 59	Able to Perform	Able to Perform with Assistance	Unable to Perform	Initials and Date
59. Comb or brush the patient's hair. *Comments:*	☐	☐	☐	
60. Apply disposable gloves and perform oral hygiene at this time. *Comments:*	☐	☐	☐	
61. Discard towels and washcloth in a laundry hamper. *Comments:*	☐	☐	☐	
62. Provide a clean gown. *Comments:*	☐	☐	☐	
63. Clean and replace equipment according to facility policy. *Comments:*	☐	☐	☐	
64. Change the bed linen, following the procedure for making an occupied bed. *Comments:*	☐	☐	☐	
65. Remove and discard disposable gloves according to facility policy. *Comments:*	☐	☐	☐	
66. Raise the side rails, if required. *Comments:*	☐	☐	☐	
67. Carry out procedure completion actions. *Comments:*	☐	☐	☐	

Checklist for Procedure 60   Changing the Patient's Gown

Name _____ Date _____

School _____

Instructor _____

Course _____

Procedure 60 Changing the Patient's Gown	Able to Perform	Able to Perform with Assistance	Unable to Perform	Initials and Date
1. Carry out beginning procedure actions. *Comments:*	☐	☐	☐	
2. Assemble equipment. *Comments:*	☐	☐	☐	
3. Place a bath blanket over the top sheet and pull the sheet down by sliding it out from under the bath blanket. *Comments:*	☐	☐	☐	
4. Loosen the gown from the patient's neck. *Comments:*	☐	☐	☐	
5. Slip the gown down the arms. *Comments:*	☐	☐	☐	
6. Make sure a bath blanket covers the patient. *Comments:*	☐	☐	☐	
7. If the patient is wearing a regular gown, remove the gown from the arm without the IV (intravenous) line and bring the gown across the patient's chest. *Comments:*	☐	☐	☐	
8. Place a clean gown over the patient's chest to avoid exposure. *Comments:*	☐	☐	☐	
9. With one hand, gather the gown on the arm with the IV so there is no pull or pressure on the IV line and slightly draw the gown over the tips of the patient's fingers. *Comments:*	☐	☐	☐	

continued on the following page

continued from the previous page

Procedure 60	Able to Perform	Able to Perform with Assistance	Unable to Perform	Initials and Date
10. With your free hand, lift the IV free of the standard and slip the gown over the bag of fluid, removing the gown from the patient's body. Never allow the bag of fluid to be lower than the patient's arm. *Comments:*	☐	☐	☐	
11. Take the sleeve of a clean gown and slip it over the bag of fluid, over the tubing, and up to the patient's arm. *Comments:*	☐	☐	☐	
12. Replace the bag of fluid on the IV standard. *Comments:*	☐	☐	☐	
13. Remove the soiled gown and place it at the end of the bed. Finish placing the clean gown on the patient's other arm. Secure the neck ties. *Comments:*	☐	☐	☐	
14. Place the soiled gown in a laundry hamper. *Comments:*	☐	☐	☐	
15. Make sure the IV is dripping at the required rate and that the tubing is not kinked or twisted. *Comments:*	☐	☐	☐	
16. If the patient has a weak or paralyzed arm, undress the patient in the following manner: a. Untie the gown and remove the back sides of the gown from beneath the patient. b. Remove the gown from the stronger arm first. c. Bring the gown across the patient's chest. d. Slide the gown down over the weak arm. e. Gently lift the patient's weak arm and finish removing the gown over the patient's head. f. Reverse the procedure to put on a clean gown. *Comments:*	☐	☐	☐	
17. Pull sheet up over the bath blanket and remove the bath blanket. *Comments:*	☐	☐	☐	
18. Carry out procedure completion actions. *Comments:*	☐	☐	☐	

Checklist for Procedure 61   Waterless Bed Bath

Name _____ Date _____

School _____

Instructor _____

Course _____

Procedure 61 **Waterless Bed Bath**	Able to **Perform**	Able to **Perform with Assistance**	**Unable to Perform**	**Initials and Date**
1. Carry out beginning procedure actions. *Comments:*	☐	☐	☐	
2. Assemble equipment. *Comments:*	☐	☐	☐	
3. Close windows and door. *Comments:*	☐	☐	☐	
4. Pull the privacy curtain. *Comments:*	☐	☐	☐	
5. Offer the bedpan or urinal. *Comments:*	☐	☐	☐	
6. Lower the head of the bed and side rail. *Comments:*	☐	☐	☐	
7. Loosen top bedclothes; remove blanket and spread. *Comments:*	☐	☐	☐	
8. Place a bath blanket over the top sheet; remove top sheet. *Comments:*	☐	☐	☐	
9. Leave one pillow under the patient's head. Place the other pillow on the chair. *Comments:*	☐	☐	☐	
10. Remove the gown and place it in a laundry hamper. *Comments:*	☐	☐	☐	
11. Assist the patient to move to the side of the bed. *Comments:*	☐	☐	☐	

continued on the following page

continued from the previous page

Procedure 61	Able to Perform	Able to Perform with Assistance	Unable to Perform	Initials and Date
12. Warm the package of waterless bathing product and apply disposable gloves. *Comments:*	☐	☐	☐	
13. Remove one cloth and cleanse the patient's face and neck. *Comments:*	☐	☐	☐	
14. Place a towel over the patient's chest. Cleanse the chest. *Comments:*	☐	☐	☐	
15. Fold the bath blanket down to the pubic area and wash the abdomen. *Comments:*	☐	☐	☐	
16. Replace the bath blanket over the chest and abdomen. *Comments:*	☐	☐	☐	
17. Wash each arm and hand. *Comments:*	☐	☐	☐	
18. Wash the axilla. *Comments:*	☐	☐	☐	
19. Apply deodorant. *Comments:*	☐	☐	☐	
20. Provide nail care as needed. *Comments:*	☐	☐	☐	
21. Expose and cleanse each leg, thigh, and foot. Cover with bath blanket. *Comments:*	☐	☐	☐	
22. Make sure the side rail on the opposite side of the bed is up. Help the patient to turn onto the side away from you. *Comments:*	☐	☐	☐	
23. Place a bath towel lengthwise next to the patient's back. *Comments:*	☐	☐	☐	

Procedure 61	Able to Perform	Able to Perform with Assistance	Unable to Perform	Initials and Date
24. Expose and wash the back and buttocks. *Comments:*	☐	☐	☐	
25. Cover the patient with the bath blanket. *Comments:*	☐	☐	☐	
26. Assist the patient to turn onto the back. *Comments:*	☐	☐	☐	
27. Place a towel under the buttocks. *Comments:*	☐	☐	☐	
28. Instruct the patient to wash the perineum. Assist if necessary. *Comments:*	☐	☐	☐	
29. Discard gloves and wash your hands. *Comments:*	☐	☐	☐	
30. Assist the patient to put on a clean gown. *Comments:*	☐	☐	☐	
31. Cover the pillow with a towel. *Comments:*	☐	☐	☐	
32. Comb and brush the patient's hair. *Comments:*	☐	☐	☐	
33. Assist with oral hygiene. *Comments:*	☐	☐	☐	
34. Change the bed linen. *Comments:*	☐	☐	☐	
35. Carry out procedure completion actions. *Comments:*	☐	☐	☐	

Checklist for Procedure 62   Partial Bath

Name _____ Date _____

School _____

Instructor _____

Course _____

Procedure 62 **Partial Bath**	Able to Perform	Able to Perform with Assistance	Unable to Perform	Initials and Date
1. Perform beginning procedure actions. *Comments:*	☐	☐	☐	
2. Assemble equipment. *Comments:*	☐	☐	☐	
3. Close the windows and door and turn off fans to prevent chilling. *Comments:*	☐	☐	☐	
4. Place towels and linens on the chair in the order of use. *Comments:*	☐	☐	☐	
5. Put on gloves. *Comments:*	☐	☐	☐	
6. Offer bedpan or urinal. *Comments:*	☐	☐	☐	
7. Elevate the head of the bed to a comfortable position. *Comments:*	☐	☐	☐	
8. Loosen the top bedclothes. Remove blanket and spread and place over the back of the chair. *Comments:*	☐	☐	☐	
9. Remove the top sheet. *Comments:*	☐	☐	☐	
10. Leave one pillow under the patient's head and place the other on a chair. *Comments:*	☐	☐	☐	

continued on the following page

continued from the previous page

Procedure 62	Able to Perform	Able to Perform with Assistance	Unable to Perform	Initials and Date
11. Assist the patient to remove the gown. Place the soiled gown in a laundry basket. *Comments:*	☐	☐	☐	
12. Cover the patient with bath blanket. *Comments:*	☐	☐	☐	
13. Place paper towels or a bed protector on the overbed table. *Comments:*	☐	☐	☐	
14. Fill a basin two-thirds full with water at 105°F and place it on the overbed table. *Comments:*	☐	☐	☐	
15. Place towels, washcloths, and soap on the overbed table comfortably close to the patient. *Comments:*	☐	☐	☐	
16. Instruct the patient to wash as much as possible and tell the patient that you will return to help complete the bath. *Comments:*	☐	☐	☐	
17. Place the call bell within easy reach. Ask the patient to call when ready. *Comments:*	☐	☐	☐	
18. Dispose of gloves, wash hands, and leave the unit. *Comments:*	☐	☐	☐	
19. When patient signals, wash hands and return to the unit. *Comments:*	☐	☐	☐	
20. Put on a pair of gloves. *Comments:*	☐	☐	☐	
21. Change the bath water. *Comments:*	☐	☐	☐	
22. Complete bathing those areas the patient could not reach. *Comments:*	☐	☐	☐	

Procedure 62	Able to Perform	Able to Perform with Assistance	Unable to Perform	Initials and Date
23. Remove gloves and discard according to facility policy. *Comments:*	☐	☐	☐	
24. Wash hands. *Comments:*	☐	☐	☐	
25. Give a backrub with lotion. *Comments:*	☐	☐	☐	
26. Assist the patient with applying deodorant and a fresh gown. *Comments:*	☐	☐	☐	
27. Cover the pillow with a towel and comb or brush hair. *Comments:*	☐	☐	☐	
28. Assist with oral hygiene. *Comments:*	☐	☐	☐	
29. Clean and replace equipment according to facility policy. *Comments:*	☐	☐	☐	
30. Place a clean washcloth and towels at bedside. *Comments:*	☐	☐	☐	
31. Change the bed linen; place soiled linen in a hamper. *Comments:*	☐	☐	☐	
32. Carry out procedure completion actions. *Comments:*	☐	☐	☐	

Checklist for Procedure 63 Female Perineal Care

Name _____ Date _____

School _____

Instructor _____

Course _____

Procedure 63 **Female Perineal Care**	Able to Perform	Able to Perform with Assistance	Unable to Perform	Initials and Date
1. Carry out beginning procedure actions. *Comments:*	☐	☐	☐	
2. Assemble equipment. *Comments:*	☐	☐	☐	
3. Lower the side rail on the side where you will be working; make certain the opposite side rail is up. *Comments:*	☐	☐	☐	
4. Remove the bedspread and blanket. Place them on the back of the chair. *Comments:*	☐	☐	☐	
5. The patient should be on her back. *Comments:*	☐	☐	☐	
6. Cover the patient with a bath blanket and fanfold the sheet to the foot of the bed. *Comments:*	☐	☐	☐	
7. Put on disposable gloves. *Comments:*	☐	☐	☐	
8. Fill the basin with water at 105°F. *Comments:*	☐	☐	☐	
9. Ask the patient to raise her hips while you place a bed protector under her. *Comments:*	☐	☐	☐	
10. Offer the bedpan. *Comments:*	☐	☐	☐	

continued on the following page

continued from the previous page

Procedure 63	Able to Perform	Able to Perform with Assistance	Unable to Perform	Initials and Date
11. Remove gloves and put on a new pair of gloves if bedpan was used. *Comments:*	☐	☐	☐	
12. Position the bath blanket so that only the area between the legs is exposed. *Comments:*	☐	☐	☐	
13. Ask the patient to separate her legs and flex her knees. *Comments:*	☐	☐	☐	
14. Wet the washcloth, make a mitt, and apply a small amount of liquid soap. *Comments:*	☐	☐	☐	
15. Stabilize and separate the vulva with one gloved hand. Using the other gloved hand, wash with one downward stroke along the far side of the outer labia to the perineum. *Comments:*	☐	☐	☐	
16. Rinse the washcloth, remake the mitt, and rinse the area just cleaned. *Comments:*	☐	☐	☐	
17. Wash the inner far labia in the same manner. *Comments:*	☐	☐	☐	
18. Wash the inner near labia. *Comments:*	☐	☐	☐	
19. With gloved hands, separate the labia. Clean and rinse the inner part of the vulva to the perineum. *Comments:*	☐	☐	☐	
20. Dry the washed area with a towel. *Comments:*	☐	☐	☐	
21. Turn the patient away from you, flexing the patient's upper leg slightly if possible. *Comments:*	☐	☐	☐	

Procedure 63	Able to Perform	Able to Perform with Assistance	Unable to Perform	Initials and Date
22. Make a mitt, wet it, and apply soap lightly. *Comments:*	☐	☐	☐	
23. Expose and wash the anal area, stroking from perineum to coccyx. *Comments:*	☐	☐	☐	
24. Rinse well. *Comments:*	☐	☐	☐	
25. Dry carefully. *Comments:*	☐	☐	☐	
26. Return the patient to her back. *Comments:*	☐	☐	☐	
27. Remove and dispose of bed protector. *Comments:*	☐	☐	☐	
28. Cover the patient with a sheet or bath blanket. *Comments:*	☐	☐	☐	
29. Remove and dispose of gloves. *Comments:*	☐	☐	☐	
30. Wash your hands. *Comments:*	☐	☐	☐	
31. Remove, fold, and store the bath blanket according to facility policy. *Comments:*	☐	☐	☐	
32. Replace the top covers, tuck them under the mattress, and make mitered corners. *Comments:*	☐	☐	☐	
33. Put up the side rail. *Comments:*	☐	☐	☐	

continued on the following page

continued from the previous page

Procedure 63	Able to Perform	Able to Perform with Assistance	Unable to Perform	Initials and Date
34. Put on gloves and empty the water. *Comments:*	☐	☐	☐	
35. Clean equipment and dispose of or store it according to facility policy. *Comments:*	☐	☐	☐	
36. Remove gloves and discard according to facility policy. *Comments:*	☐	☐	☐	
37. Wash your hands. *Comments:*	☐	☐	☐	
38. Carry out procedure completion actions. *Comments:*	☐	☐	☐	

Checklist for Procedure 64   Male Perineal Care

Name _____ Date _____

School _____

Instructor _____

Course _____

Procedure 64 Male Perineal Care	Able to Perform	Able to Perform with Assistance	Unable to Perform	Initials and Date
1. Carry out beginning procedure actions. *Comments:*	☐	☐	☐	
2. Assemble your equipment. *Comments:*	☐	☐	☐	
3. Fill a basin with warm water (approximately 105°F). *Comments:*	☐	☐	☐	
4. Lower the rail on the side of the bed where you will be working. *Comments:*	☐	☐	☐	
5. Fanfold the blanket and spread to the foot of the bed. *Comments:*	☐	☐	☐	
6. Remove, fold, and place blanket and spread on the back of the chair. *Comments:*	☐	☐	☐	
7. Cover the patient with a bath blanket and fanfold the sheet to the foot of the bed. *Comments:*	☐	☐	☐	
8. Put on disposable gloves. *Comments:*	☐	☐	☐	
9. Place a bed protector under the patient's buttocks. *Comments:*	☐	☐	☐	
10. Offer the bedpan or urinal. *Comments:*	☐	☐	☐	
11. Have the patient flex and separate his knees. *Comments:*	☐	☐	☐	

continued on the following page

continued from the previous page

Procedure 64	Able to Perform	Able to Perform with Assistance	Unable to Perform	Initials and Date
12. Draw the bath blanket upward to expose the perineal area only. *Comments:*	☐	☐	☐	
13. Make a mitt with a washcloth and apply a small amount of soap. *Comments:*	☐	☐	☐	
14. Grasp the penis gently with one hand and wash, in a circular motion, beginning at the meatus. If the patient is not circumcised, draw back the foreskin. *Comments:*	☐	☐	☐	
15. Rinse thoroughly. *Comments:*	☐	☐	☐	
16. Continue to wash down the penis and the rest of the perineal area, including the scrotum, using downward strokes and working outward to thighs. *Comments:*	☐	☐	☐	
17. Lift the scrotum and wash the perineum. *Comments:*	☐	☐	☐	
18. Rinse the washcloth and remake a mitt. *Comments:*	☐	☐	☐	
19. Rinse the urethral and perineal areas well, working in the same direction until the entire area is clean and soap-free. *Comments:*	☐	☐	☐	
20. Dry the washed area with a towel. *Comments:*	☐	☐	☐	
21. Reposition the foreskin, if necessary. *Comments:*	☐	☐	☐	
22. Turn the patient away from you. *Comments:*	☐	☐	☐	
23. Make a mitt, wet it, and apply soap lightly. *Comments:*	☐	☐	☐	
24. Expose and wash the anal area, stroking from perineum to coccyx. *Comments:*	☐	☐	☐	

Procedure 64	Able to Perform	Able to Perform with Assistance	Unable to Perform	Initials and Date
25. Rinse well. *Comments:*	☐	☐	☐	
26. Dry carefully. *Comments:*	☐	☐	☐	
27. Return the patient to his back. *Comments:*	☐	☐	☐	
28. Remove and dispose of gloves according to facility policy. *Comments:*	☐	☐	☐	
29. Wash your hands. *Comments:*	☐	☐	☐	
30. Remove, fold, and store the bath blanket, according to facility policy. *Comments:*	☐	☐	☐	
31. Replace the top covers, tuck them under the mattress, and make mitered corners. *Comments:*	☐	☐	☐	
32. Raise the side rail, if required. *Comments:*	☐	☐	☐	
33. Put on gloves. *Comments:*	☐	☐	☐	
34. Empty the water. *Comments:*	☐	☐	☐	
35. Clean equipment and dispose of or store it according to facility policy. *Comments:*	☐	☐	☐	
36. Remove gloves and discard according to facility policy. *Comments:*	☐	☐	☐	
37. Wash your hands. *Comments:*	☐	☐	☐	
38. Carry out procedure completion actions. *Comments:*	☐	☐	☐	

Checklist for Procedure 65   Hand and Fingernail Care

Name _____ Date _____

School _____

Instructor _____

Course _____

Procedure 65 Hand and Fingernail Care	Able to Perform	Able to Perform with Assistance	Unable to Perform	Initials and Date
1. Carry out beginning procedure actions. *Comments:*	☐	☐	☐	
2. Assemble equipment. *Comments:*	☐	☐	☐	
3. Elevate the head of the bed or, if the patient is allowed out of bed, transfer the patient to a chair. *Comments:*	☐	☐	☐	
4. Position the overbed table in front of the patient. *Comments:*	☐	☐	☐	
5. Place a plastic protector on the overbed table. *Comments:*	☐	☐	☐	
6. Fill a basin with warm water at approximately 105°F; then place it on the overbed table. *Comments:*	☐	☐	☐	
7. Instruct the patient to put hands in basin and soak for approximately 5 minutes. *Comments:*	☐	☐	☐	
8. Place a towel over basin to retain heat. *Comments:*	☐	☐	☐	
9. Wash the patient's hands. *Comments:*	☐	☐	☐	
10. Push cuticles back gently with a washcloth or an orangewood stick. *Comments:*	☐	☐	☐	

continued on the following page

continued from the previous page

Procedure 65	Able to Perform	Able to Perform with Assistance	Unable to Perform	Initials and Date
11. Clean under the nails. *Comments:*	☐	☐	☐	
12. Dry the patient's hands with a towel. *Comments:*	☐	☐	☐	
13. Use nail clippers to cut fingernails straight across. *Comments:*	☐	☐	☐	
14. Shape and smooth the fingernails with an emery board. *Comments:*	☐	☐	☐	
15. Pour a small amount of lotion in your palms and gently smooth it on the patient's hands. *Comments:*	☐	☐	☐	
16. Empty the basin of water. *Comments:*	☐	☐	☐	
17. Gather equipment. *Comments:*	☐	☐	☐	
18. Clean and store equipment according to facility policy. *Comments:*	☐	☐	☐	
19. Return the overbed table to the foot of the bed. *Comments:*	☐	☐	☐	
20. Return the patient to bed, if necessary. *Comments:*	☐	☐	☐	
21. Carry out procedure completion actions. *Comments:*	☐	☐	☐	

Checklist for Procedure 66   Bed Shampoo

Name _____ Date _____

School _____

Instructor _____

Course _____

Procedure 66 Bed Shampoo	Able to Perform	Able to Perform with Assistance	Unable to Perform	Initials and Date
1. Carry out beginning procedure actions. *Comments:*	☐	☐	☐	
2. Assemble equipment. *Comments:*	☐	☐	☐	
3. Place a large, empty basin on the floor under the spout of the shampoo tray. *Comments:*	☐	☐	☐	
4. Arrange equipment on bedstand. *Comments:*	☐	☐	☐	
5. Replace top bedding with a bath blanket. *Comments:*	☐	☐	☐	
6. Ask the patient to move to the side of the bed nearest you. Assist as needed. *Comments:*	☐	☐	☐	
7. Replace the pillowcase with a waterproof covering. *Comments:*	☐	☐	☐	
8. Cover the head of the bed with a bed protector, making sure it extends under the patient's shoulders. *Comments:*	☐	☐	☐	
9. Loosen neck ties of gown. *Comments:*	☐	☐	☐	
10. Place a towel under the patient's head and shoulders. *Comments:*	☐	☐	☐	
11. Brush hair free of tangles, working snarls out carefully. *Comments:*	☐	☐	☐	

continued on the following page

continued from the previous page

Procedure 66	Able to Perform	Able to Perform with Assistance	Unable to Perform	Initials and Date
12. Bring the towel down around the patient's neck and shoulders and pin it. *Comments:*	☐	☐	☐	
13. Position the pillow under shoulders so that the patient's head is tilted slightly backward. *Comments:*	☐	☐	☐	
14. Raise the bed to a high horizontal position. *Comments:*	☐	☐	☐	
15. Raise the patient's head and position the shampoo tray so that the drain is over the edge of the bed directly above the basin. *Comments:*	☐	☐	☐	
16. Give the patient a washcloth to cover eyes. *Comments:*	☐	☐	☐	
17. Recheck water temperature. *Comments:*	☐	☐	☐	
18. Using a small pitcher, pour a small amount of water over hair until thoroughly wet. Use one hand to direct the flow away from the face and ears. *Comments:*	☐	☐	☐	
19. Apply a small amount of shampoo, working up a lather. *Comments:*	☐	☐	☐	
20. Massage the scalp with your fingertips. Avoid using your fingernails. *Comments:*	☐	☐	☐	
21. Rinse thoroughly, pouring from hairline to hair tips. *Comments:*	☐	☐	☐	
22. Repeat lathering and rinsing. *Comments:*	☐	☐	☐	
23. Lift the patient's head to remove the tray and bed protector. *Comments:*	☐	☐	☐	

Procedure 66	Able to Perform	Able to Perform with Assistance	Unable to Perform	Initials and Date
24. Adjust the pillow and slip a dry bath towel underneath the head. *Comments:*	☐	☐	☐	
25. Place the tray on the basin. *Comments:*	☐	☐	☐	
26. Wrap hair in a towel, drying face, neck, and ears as needed. *Comments:*	☐	☐	☐	
27. Dry hair with towel or a dryer as indicated. *Comments:*	☐	☐	☐	
28. Comb the hair appropriately. *Comments:*	☐	☐	☐	
29. Remove the protective pillow cover; replace with a cloth cover. *Comments:*	☐	☐	☐	
30. Lower the bed to a comfortable working position. *Comments:*	☐	☐	☐	
31. Replace the bedding and remove the bath blanket. *Comments:*	☐	☐	☐	
32. Help the patient assume a comfortable position. *Comments:*	☐	☐	☐	
33. Lower the bed to the lowest horizontal position. *Comments:*	☐	☐	☐	
34. Leave the call bell within reach. *Comments:*	☐	☐	☐	
35. Allow the patient to rest undisturbed. *Comments:*	☐	☐	☐	
36. Empty the water from the collection basin. *Comments:*	☐	☐	☐	
37. Carry out procedure completion actions. *Comments:*	☐	☐	☐	

Checklist for Procedure 67   Dressing and Undressing the Patient

Name _____ Date _____

School _____

Instructor _____

Course _____

Procedure 67 Dressing and Undressing the Patient	Able to Perform	Able to Perform with Assistance	Unable to Perform	Initials and Date
1. Carry out beginning procedure actions. *Comments:*	☐	☐	☐	
2. Select appropriate clothing and arrange in order of application. *Comments:*	☐	☐	☐	
3. Cover the patient with a bath blanket and fanfold top bedclothes to foot of bed. *Comments:*	☐	☐	☐	
4. Elevate the head of the bed to a sitting position. *Comments:*	☐	☐	☐	
5. Assist the patient to a comfortable sitting position. *Comments:*	☐	☐	☐	
6. Remove night clothing beginning with the strong side first and then the weaker side. *Comments:*	☐	☐	☐	
7. If the patient wears a bra, slip the straps over the patient's hands (weak side first), move the straps up her arms, and position them on her shoulders. *Comments:*	☐	☐	☐	
8. For any garment that slips over the head, gather the garment and place it over the patient's head. *Comments:*	☐	☐	☐	
9. Grasp the patient's hand and guide it through the armhole by reaching into the armhole from the outside. *Comments:*	☐	☐	☐	
10. Repeat the procedure with the opposite arm. *Comments:*	☐	☐	☐	

continued on the following page

continued from the previous page

Procedure 67	Able to Perform	Able to Perform with Assistance	Unable to Perform	Initials and Date
11. Assist the patient to lean forward and adjust the garment so it is smooth over the body. *Comments:*	☐	☐	☐	
12. For shirts or dresses that fasten in front, insert your hand through the sleeve of the garment and grasp the patient's hand. *Comments:*	☐	☐	☐	
13. Draw the sleeve over your hand and the patient's. *Comments:*	☐	☐	☐	
14. Adjust the sleeve at the shoulder. *Comments:*	☐	☐	☐	
15. Assist the patient to sit forward and arrange clothing across the patient's back. *Comments:*	☐	☐	☐	
16. Gather the sleeve on the opposite side by slipping your hand in from the inside. *Comments:*	☐	☐	☐	
17. Grasp the patient's wrist and pull the sleeve of the garment over your hand and the patient's hand. *Comments:*	☐	☐	☐	
18. Draw the sleeve upward and adjust it at the shoulder. *Comments:*	☐	☐	☐	
19. Button, zip, or snap the garment. *Comments:*	☐	☐	☐	
20. For underwear or pants, face the bed and gather the patient's underwear from waist to leg hole. *Comments:*	☐	☐	☐	
21. Slip the underwear over one foot at a time; pull underwear up legs as high as possible. *Comments:*	☐	☐	☐	
22. Assist the patient to raise the hips. *Comments:*	☐	☐	☐	

Procedure 67	Able to Perform	Able to Perform with Assistance	Unable to Perform	Initials and Date
23. Draw the garment over the buttocks and up to the waist. Adjust until comfortable. *Comments:*	☐	☐	☐	
24. Fasten the garment, if required. *Comments:*	☐	☐	☐	
25. For stockings or socks, roll with heel in back and place it over the toes. *Comments:*	☐	☐	☐	
26. Draw the sock up over the foot and adjust until smooth. *Comments:*	☐	☐	☐	
27. Pull stockings up to knee or thigh. *Comments:*	☐	☐	☐	
28. Repeat for other foot. *Comments:*	☐	☐	☐	
29. For pantyhose, gather them and adjust over toes and feet. *Comments:*	☐	☐	☐	
30. Draw up legs as high as possible. *Comments:*	☐	☐	☐	
31. Assist the patient to raise the hips and draw over hips. *Comments:*	☐	☐	☐	
32. Adjust until comfortable. *Comments:*	☐	☐	☐	
33. For shoes, open the laces of the shoe completely and slip the shoe on. *Comments:*	☐	☐	☐	
34. Ensure that the shoe is fastened securely. *Comments:*	☐	☐	☐	
35. To undress, reverse order of steps. *Comments:*	☐	☐	☐	
36. Carry out procedure completion actions. *Comments:*	☐	☐	☐	

Checklist for Procedure 68 Assisting with Routine Oral Hygiene

Name _____ Date _____

School _____

Instructor _____

Course _____

Procedure 68 **Assisting with Routine Oral Hygiene**	Able to Perform	Able to Perform with Assistance	Unable to Perform	Initials and Date
1. Carry out beginning procedure actions. *Comments:*	☐	☐	☐	
2. Assemble equipment. *Comments:*	☐	☐	☐	
3. Raise the head of the bed. *Comments:*	☐	☐	☐	
4. Lower the side rails. *Comments:*	☐	☐	☐	
5. Position the overbed table across the patient's lap and cover with a protector. *Comments:*	☐	☐	☐	
6. Place equipment on the table. *Comments:*	☐	☐	☐	
7. Place a bath towel over the patient's gown and bedcovers. *Comments:*	☐	☐	☐	
8. Be prepared to help where necessary. *Comments:*	☐	☐	☐	
9. Pour water over the toothbrush. *Comments:*	☐	☐	☐	
10. Put toothpaste on the brush. *Comments:*	☐	☐	☐	
11. Apply disposable gloves. *Comments:*	☐	☐	☐	

continued on the following page

continued from the previous page

Procedure 68	Able to Perform	Able to Perform with Assistance	Unable to Perform	Initials and Date
12. Insert the toothbrush into the mouth with bristles pointing downward. *Comments:*	☐	☐	☐	
13. Turn the toothbrush with bristles toward the teeth. *Comments:*	☐	☐	☐	
14. Brush all tooth surfaces with a back-and-forth motion, using short strokes. *Comments:*	☐	☐	☐	
15. Use the toe end of the brush to clean the inner surfaces of the front teeth, using a gentle up-and-down motion. *Comments:*	☐	☐	☐	
16. Brush the front of the tongue gently, if tolerated by the patient. *Comments:*	☐	☐	☐	
17. Give the patient a cup of water to rinse the mouth. *Comments:*	☐	☐	☐	
18. Turn the patient's head to one side, with an emesis basin near the chin, for return of fluid. *Comments:*	☐	☐	☐	
19. Repeat rinsing as necessary. *Comments:*	☐	☐	☐	
20. Select a piece of dental floss about 12 inches long. *Comments:*	☐	☐	☐	
21. Wrap the end of the floss around your middle fingers, leaving the center area free. *Comments:*	☐	☐	☐	
22. Ask the patient to open her mouth. *Comments:*	☐	☐	☐	
23. Gently insert the floss between each tooth down to, but not into, the gum line. *Comments:*	☐	☐	☐	

Procedure 68	Able to Perform	Able to Perform with Assistance	Unable to Perform	Initials and Date
24. Ask the patient to rinse her mouth using the emesis basin. *Comments:*	☐	☐	☐	
25. Offer the patient mouthwash. Dilute if the patient wishes. *Comments:*	☐	☐	☐	
26. Remove the basin. *Comments:*	☐	☐	☐	
27. Wipe the patient's mouth and chin with tissue. *Comments:*	☐	☐	☐	
28. Discard the tissue in a paper bag. *Comments:*	☐	☐	☐	
29. Remove the towel. *Comments:*	☐	☐	☐	
30. Rinse the toothbrush with water. *Comments:*	☐	☐	☐	
31. Remove and dispose of gloves. *Comments:*	☐	☐	☐	
32. Carry out procedure completion actions. *Comments:*	☐	☐	☐	

Checklist for Procedure 69   Assisting with Special Oral Hygiene

Name _____ Date _____

School _____

Instructor _____

Course _____

Procedure 69 **Assisting with Special Oral Hygiene**	Able to Perform	Able to Perform with Assistance	Unable to Perform	Initials and Date
1. Carry out beginning procedure actions. *Comments:*	☐	☐	☐	
2. Assemble equipment. *Comments:*	☐	☐	☐	
3. Apply disposable gloves. *Comments:*	☐	☐	☐	
4. Cover the pillow with a towel. *Comments:*	☐	☐	☐	
5. Elevate the head of the bed, if patient is able to sit up. *Comments:*	☐	☐	☐	
6. If the patient is not able to sit up, turn the patient's head to one side and slightly forward. *Comments:*	☐	☐	☐	
7. Cover the patient's upper chest with a towel. *Comments:*	☐	☐	☐	
8. Place an emesis basin under the patient's chin. *Comments:*	☐	☐	☐	
9. Gently pull down on the chin to open the mouth, or open the mouth gently with a tongue depressor. *Comments:*	☐	☐	☐	
10. Using moistened Toothettes®, wipe gums, teeth, tongue, and inside of mouth. *Comments:*	☐	☐	☐	

continued on the following page

continued from the previous page

Procedure 69	Able to Perform	Able to Perform with Assistance	Unable to Perform	Initials and Date
11. Discard used applicators in a plastic bag. *Comments:*	☐	☐	☐	
12. Apply lubricant to the patient's lips with a clean applicator. *Comments:*	☐	☐	☐	
13. Place used applicators in a plastic bag. *Comments:*	☐	☐	☐	
14. Remove towels. *Comments:*	☐	☐	☐	
15. Clean and replace equipment. *Comments:*	☐	☐	☐	
16. Remove and dispose of gloves. *Comments:*	☐	☐	☐	
17. Wash your hands. *Comments:*	☐	☐	☐	
18. Carry out procedure completion actions. *Comments:*	☐	☐	☐	

Checklist for Procedure 70 Assisting the Patient to Floss and Brush Teeth

Name _____ Date _____

School _____

Instructor _____

Course _____

Procedure 70 **Assisting the Patient to Floss and Brush Teeth**	Able to Perform	Able to Perform with Assistance	Unable to Perform	Initials and Date
1. Carry out beginning procedure actions. *Comments:*	☐	☐	☐	
2. Assemble equipment. *Comments:*	☐	☐	☐	
3. Elevate the head of the bed and help the patient into a comfortable position. *Comments:*	☐	☐	☐	
4. Lower the side rails. *Comments:*	☐	☐	☐	
5. Position the overbed table across the patient's lap. *Comments:*	☐	☐	☐	
6. Cover the table with a plastic protector. *Comments:*	☐	☐	☐	
7. Place an emesis basin and a glass of water on the overbed table. *Comments:*	☐	☐	☐	
8. Place a towel across the patient's chest. *Comments:*	☐	☐	☐	
9. Be prepared to help as the patient flosses and brushes teeth. *Comments:*	☐	☐	☐	
10. Remind the patient to clean the tongue and gums. *Comments:*	☐	☐	☐	

continued on the following page

continued from the previous page

Procedure 70	Able to Perform	Able to Perform with Assistance	Unable to Perform	Initials and Date
11. Apply disposable gloves. *Comments:*	☐	☐	☐	
12. If assisting with the procedure, use standard precautions. *Comments:*	☐	☐	☐	
13. After patient is finished, push the overbed table to the foot of the bed. *Comments:*	☐	☐	☐	
14. Remove the emesis basin. *Comments:*	☐	☐	☐	
15. Clean the basin and replace it according to facility policy. *Comments:*	☐	☐	☐	
16. Rinse toothbrush. *Comments:*	☐	☐	☐	
17. Remove the towels and put them with the soiled linen. *Comments:*	☐	☐	☐	
18. Remove gloves and discard. *Comments:*	☐	☐	☐	
19. Carry out procedure completion actions. *Comments:*	☐	☐	☐	

Checklist for Procedure 71   Caring for Dentures

Name _____ Date _____

School _____

Instructor _____

Course _____

Procedure 71 **Caring for Dentures**	Able to Perform	Able to Perform with Assistance	Unable to Perform	Initials and Date
1. Carry out beginning procedure actions. *Comments:*	☐	☐	☐	
2. Assemble equipment. *Comments:*	☐	☐	☐	
3. Apply disposable gloves. *Comments:*	☐	☐	☐	
4. Allow the patient to clean the dentures if she is able to do so. *Comments:*	☐	☐	☐	
5. If the patient is unable to clean the dentures, give her a tissue and ask her to remove the dentures. *Comments:*	☐	☐	☐	
6. If assistance is necessary, grasp the upper dentures firmly. *Comments:*	☐	☐	☐	
7. Ease the dentures downward and then forward, and remove them from the mouth. *Comments:*	☐	☐	☐	
8. Grasp the lower dentures firmly, ease them upward and then forward, and remove them from the mouth. *Comments:*	☐	☐	☐	
9. Place the dentures in a denture cup padded with gauze squares. *Comments:*	☐	☐	☐	
10. Take the dentures to the bathroom or utility room. *Comments:*	☐	☐	☐	

continued on the following page

continued from the previous page

Procedure 71	Able to Perform	Able to Perform with Assistance	Unable to Perform	Initials and Date
11. Place a paper towel or washcloth in the bottom of the basin. *Comments:*	☐	☐	☐	
12. Fill the sink half full with cold water. *Comments:*	☐	☐	☐	
13. Soak the dentures in a solution with a cleansing tablet before brushing, if desired. *Comments:*	☐	☐	☐	
14. Rinse the dentures under cool water. *Comments:*	☐	☐	☐	
15. Put toothpaste or tooth powder on a brush. *Comments:*	☐	☐	☐	
16. Hold the dentures and brush until all surfaces are clean. *Comments:*	☐	☐	☐	
17. Rinse the dentures thoroughly under cool or warm running water. Never use hot water. *Comments:*	☐	☐	☐	
18. Rinse the denture cup. *Comments:*	☐	☐	☐	
19. Place fresh gauze squares in the denture cup with clean, cool water. *Comments:*	☐	☐	☐	
20. Place the dentures in the gauze-lined cup and take them to the bedside. *Comments:*	☐	☐	☐	
21. Assist the patient to rinse her mouth with water or mouthwash, if permitted. *Comments:*	☐	☐	☐	

Procedure 71	Able to Perform	Able to Perform with Assistance	Unable to Perform	Initials and Date
22. Hold the mouth open gently with a wooden tongue depressor. *Comments:*	☐	☐	☐	
23. Clean the gums and tongue with applicators moistened with mouthwash or use Toothettes®. *Comments:*	☐	☐	☐	
24. Hand wet dentures to the patient using a paper towel or gauze. *Comments:*	☐	☐	☐	
25. If the patient is able, she may remove the dentures from the cup. *Comments:*	☐	☐	☐	
26. If assistance is needed, insert first the upper denture then the lower. *Comments:*	☐	☐	☐	
27. Clean and replace equipment. *Comments:*	☐	☐	☐	
28. Remove and dispose of gloves. *Comments:*	☐	☐	☐	
29. Carry out procedure completion actions. *Comments:*	☐	☐	☐	

Checklist for Procedure 72   Backrub

Name _____ Date _____

School _____

Instructor _____

Course _____

Procedure 72 Backrub	Able to Perform	Able to Perform with Assistance	Unable to Perform	Initials and Date
1. Carry out beginning procedure actions. Comments:	☐	☐	☐	
2. Assemble equipment. Comments:	☐	☐	☐	
3. Put up the far side rail of the bed. Comments:	☐	☐	☐	
4. Warm lotion in a basin of water. Comments:	☐	☐	☐	
5. Apply gloves if patient has open lesions. Comments:	☐	☐	☐	
6. Turn the patient on his side with the back toward you. Comments:	☐	☐	☐	
7. Expose and wash the back. This step in unnecessary if a backrub is given after a bath. Comments:	☐	☐	☐	
8. Dry carefully. Comments:	☐	☐	☐	
9. Pour a small amount of lotion into one hand and warm it in the palm of your hand. Comments:	☐	☐	☐	
10. Apply the lotion to the patient's skin and rub with gentle but firm strokes. Comments:	☐	☐	☐	

continued on the following page

continued from the previous page

Procedure 72	Able to Perform	Able to Perform with Assistance	Unable to Perform	Initials and Date
11. Give special attention to all bony prominences. *Comments:*	☐	☐	☐	
12. Do not rub red areas. Report these to the nurse. *Comments:*	☐	☐	☐	
13. Begin at the base of the spine and use long, soothing strokes. *Comments:*	☐	☐	☐	
14. Rub up the center of the back, around the shoulders, and down the sides of the back and buttocks; repeat four times. Use soothing upward strokes and a circular motion on the downstroke. *Comments:*	☐	☐	☐	
15. Repeat, but on the downward stroke rub in small circular motions with the palm of your hand. Include areas over the coccyx. *Comments:*	☐	☐	☐	
16. Repeat long, soothing strokes on muscles for 3 to 5 minutes. *Comments:*	☐	☐	☐	
17. Dry the area well. *Comments:*	☐	☐	☐	
18. Report any redness on pressure areas to the nurse. *Comments:*	☐	☐	☐	
19. Straighten and tighten the bottom sheet and draw sheet. *Comments:*	☐	☐	☐	
20. Change the patient's gown, if necessary. *Comments:*	☐	☐	☐	
21. Remove and dispose of gloves. *Comments:*	☐	☐	☐	
22. Replace equipment. *Comments:*	☐	☐	☐	
23. Carry out procedure completion actions. *Comments:*	☐	☐	☐	

Checklist for Procedure 73   Shaving a Male Patient

Name _____ Date _____

School _____

Instructor _____

Course _____

Procedure 73 Shaving a Male Patient	Able to Perform	Able to Perform with Assistance	Unable to Perform	Initials and Date
1. Carry out beginning procedure actions. *Comments:*	☐	☐	☐	
2. Assemble equipment. *Comments:*	☐	☐	☐	
3. Raise the head of the bed. *Comments:*	☐	☐	☐	
4. Place equipment on the overbed table. *Comments:*	☐	☐	☐	
5. Apply disposable gloves. *Comments:*	☐	☐	☐	
6. Place one face towel across the patient's chest and one under the head. *Comments:*	☐	☐	☐	
7. Moisten the face and apply lather. *Comments:*	☐	☐	☐	
8. Starting in front of the ear, hold skin taunt and bring razor down over cheek toward chin. *Comments:*	☐	☐	☐	
9. Repeat until lather on cheek is removed and the area has been shaved. *Comments:*	☐	☐	☐	
10. Rinse frequently. *Comments:*	☐	☐	☐	

continued on the following page

continued from the previous page

Procedure 73	Able to Perform	Able to Perform with Assistance	Unable to Perform	Initials and Date
11. Repeat on other cheek. *Comments:*	☐	☐	☐	
12. Use firm, short strokes and shave in direction of hair growth. *Comments:*	☐	☐	☐	
13. Rinse razor frequently. *Comments:*	☐	☐	☐	
14. Ask the patient to tighten his upper lip. *Comments:*	☐	☐	☐	
15. Shave from the nose to the upper lip in short, downward stokes. *Comments:*	☐	☐	☐	
16. Ask the patient to tighten his chin. *Comments:*	☐	☐	☐	
17. Shave the chin in downward stokes. *Comments:*	☐	☐	☐	
18. Assist the patient to tip his head back. *Comments:*	☐	☐	☐	
19. Lather the neck area and stroke up toward the chin. *Comments:*	☐	☐	☐	
20. Rinse and repeat until all lather is removed. *Comments:*	☐	☐	☐	
21. Wash the patient's face and neck and dry thoroughly. *Comments:*	☐	☐	☐	
22. Apply aftershave lotion if the patient desires. *Comments:*	☐	☐	☐	
23. If the skin is nicked, apply a small piece of tissue and hold pressure directly over the area. *Comments:*	☐	☐	☐	

Procedure 73	Able to Perform	Able to Perform with Assistance	Unable to Perform	Initials and Date
24. Apply antiseptic and bandage. Report incidence to the nurse. *Comments:*	☐	☐	☐	
25. Clean and replace equipment. *Comments:*	☐	☐	☐	
26. Dispose of razor according to policy. *Comments:*	☐	☐	☐	
27. Remove the head of an electric razor and use a razor brush to remove drippings. *Comments:*	☐	☐	☐	
28. Store razor according to policy. *Comments:*	☐	☐	☐	
29. Remove and dispose of gloves. *Comments:*	☐	☐	☐	
30. Carry out procedure completion actions. *Comments:*	☐	☐	☐	

Checklist for Procedure 74   Daily Hair Care

Name _____ Date _____

School _____

Instructor _____

Course _____

Procedure 74 Daily Hair Care	Able to Perform	Able to Perform with Assistance	Unable to Perform	Initials and Date
1. Carry out beginning procedure actions. *Comments:*	☐	☐	☐	
2. Assemble equipment. *Comments:*	☐	☐	☐	
3. Ask the patient to move to the side of the bed nearest you, or the patient may sit in a chair if permitted. *Comments:*	☐	☐	☐	
4. If the patient is sitting up, place a towel around her shoulders. *Comments:*	☐	☐	☐	
5. Cover the pillow with a towel. *Comments:*	☐	☐	☐	
6. Part or section the hair and comb with one hand between the scalp and the ends of the hair. *Comments:*	☐	☐	☐	
7. Brush carefully and thoroughly. *Comments:*	☐	☐	☐	
8. Have the patient turn so that you can comb and brush the hair on the back of her head. *Comments:*	☐	☐	☐	
9. If the hair is tangled, work section by section to unsnarl it, beginning near the ends and working toward the scalp. *Comments:*	☐	☐	☐	
10. Complete brushing and arrange the hair attractively, allowing the patient to choose the style, if able. *Comments:*	☐	☐	☐	

continued on the following page

continued from the previous page

Procedure 74	Able to Perform	Able to Perform with Assistance	Unable to Perform	Initials and Date
11. Braid long hair to prevent repeated snarling. *Comments:*	☐	☐	☐	
12. Clean and replace equipment. *Comments:*	☐	☐	☐	
13. Carry out procedure completion actions. *Comments:*	☐	☐	☐	

Checklist for Procedure 75   Giving and Receiving the Bedpan

Name _____ Date _____

School _____

Instructor _____

Course _____

Procedure 75 Giving and Receiving the Bedpan	Able to Perform	Able to Perform with Assistance	Unable to Perform	Initials and Date
1. Carry out beginning procedure actions. *Comments:*	☐	☐	☐	
2. Assemble equipment. *Comments:*	☐	☐	☐	
3. Lower the head of the bed. *Comments:*	☐	☐	☐	
4. Apply disposable gloves. *Comments:*	☐	☐	☐	
5. Take the bedpan and toilet tissue from the bedside stand. *Comments:*	☐	☐	☐	
6. Place a protector on the chair and place the bedpan on it. *Comments:*	☐	☐	☐	
7. Place the remainder of the items on the bedside table. *Comments:*	☐	☐	☐	
8. Place the bedpan cover at the foot of the bed. *Comments:*	☐	☐	☐	
9. Warm the bedpan if necessary by running warm water into it; empty and dry. *Comments:*	☐	☐	☐	
10. Cover the patient with a bath blanket. *Comments:*	☐	☐	☐	
11. Fold the top bedcovers back at a right angle. *Comments:*	☐	☐	☐	

continued on the following page

continued from the previous page

Procedure 75	Able to Perform	Able to Perform with Assistance	Unable to Perform	Initials and Date
12. Raise the patient's gown. *Comments:*	☐	☐	☐	
13. Ask the patient to flex the knees and rest weight on the heels, if able. *Comments:*	☐	☐	☐	
14. Help the patient to raise the buttocks by putting one hand under the small of the patient's back and lifting gently and slowly. *Comments:*	☐	☐	☐	
15. With the other hand, place the bedpan under the patient's hips. *Comments:*	☐	☐	☐	
16. If the patient is unable to lift the buttocks, two assistants may be needed. *Comments:*	☐	☐	☐	
17. The pan may also be placed by rolling the patient to one side. *Comments:*	☐	☐	☐	
18. Position the pan against the buttocks and roll the patient back onto the pan. *Comments:*	☐	☐	☐	
19. Check to be sure that the bedpan is positioned properly. *Comments:*	☐	☐	☐	
20. If a trapeze is in place over the bed, place the bedpan under the patient as the patient lifts himself using the trapeze. *Comments:*	☐	☐	☐	
21. Replace the top bedcovers. *Comments:*	☐	☐	☐	
22. Raise the head of the bed to a comfortable height. *Comments:*	☐	☐	☐	

Procedure 75	Able to Perform	Able to Perform with Assistance	Unable to Perform	Initials and Date
23. Remove and dispose of gloves. *Comments:*	☐	☐	☐	
24. Place toilet paper and signal cord within easy reach of the patient. *Comments:*	☐	☐	☐	
25. Leave the patient alone unless contraindicated in the nursing care plan. *Comments:*	☐	☐	☐	
26. Wash your hands. *Comments:*	☐	☐	☐	
27. Watch for the patient's signal and answer his call immediately. *Comments:*	☐	☐	☐	
28. Wash your hands and apply disposable gloves. *Comments:*	☐	☐	☐	
29. Fill the basin with warm water and place it next to the soap, washcloth, and towel on the overbed table. *Comments:*	☐	☐	☐	
30. Fold the top bedcovers back so that the patient remains covered only with the bath blanket. *Comments:*	☐	☐	☐	
31. Ask the patient to flex the knees and rest weight on the heels. *Comments:*	☐	☐	☐	
32. Place one hand under the small of the back and lift gently. *Comments:*	☐	☐	☐	
33. Remove the bedpan with the other hand. *Comments:*	☐	☐	☐	
34. Cover the bedpan and place it on the chair. *Comments:*	☐	☐	☐	

continued on the following page

continued from the previous page

Procedure 75	Able to Perform	Able to Perform with Assistance	Unable to Perform	Initials and Date
35. If the patient is unable to raise the buttocks, roll the patient off the pan to the side and remove the pan. *Comments:*	☐	☐	☐	
36. Hold the bedpan firmly with one hand, lift it, and remove. *Comments:*	☐	☐	☐	
37. If necessary, provide perineal care. *Comments:*	☐	☐	☐	
38. Discard used toilet tissue in the bedpan and cover the pan. *Comments:*	☐	☐	☐	
39. Cleanse the patient with warm water and soap, if necessary. *Comments:*	☐	☐	☐	
40. Replace the bedclothes. *Comments:*	☐	☐	☐	
41. Change linen or protective pads, if necessary. *Comments:*	☐	☐	☐	
42. Cover the patient with top bedding and remove bath blanket. *Comments:*	☐	☐	☐	
43. Encourage the patient to wash hands and freshen up. *Comments:*	☐	☐	☐	
44. Take the bedpan to the bathroom or utility room and observe contents. *Comments:*	☐	☐	☐	
45. Measure contents if required. *Comments:*	☐	☐	☐	
46. Empty the bedpan. *Comments:*	☐	☐	☐	

Procedure 75	Able to Perform	Able to Perform with Assistance	Unable to Perform	Initials and Date
47. Turn on the faucet using a paper towel. *Comments:*	☐	☐	☐	
48. Rinse the bedpan with cold water and disinfectant. *Comments:*	☐	☐	☐	
49. Rinse, dry, and return the bedpan to storage in the patient's bedside stand. *Comments:*	☐	☐	☐	
50. Remove and dispose of gloves. *Comments:*	☐	☐	☐	
51. Wash your hands. *Comments:*	☐	☐	☐	
52. Carry out procedure completion actions. *Comments:*	☐	☐	☐	
53. Empty unless you observe anything unusual. If so, save the contents for the nurse to inspect. *Comments:*	☐	☐	☐	

Checklist for Procedure 76   Giving and Receiving the Urinal

Name _____ Date _____

School _____

Instructor _____

Course _____

Procedure 76 Giving and Receiving the Urinal	Able to Perform	Able to Perform with Assistance	Unable to Perform	Initials and Date
1. Carry out beginning procedure actions. *Comments:*	☐	☐	☐	
2. Assemble equipment. *Comments:*	☐	☐	☐	
3. Apply disposable gloves. *Comments:*	☐	☐	☐	
4. Lift the bedcovers and place the urinal under the covers so the patient can grasp the handle. *Comments:*	☐	☐	☐	
5. Instruct the patient to place his penis in the urinal opening; assist if necessary. *Comments:*	☐	☐	☐	
6. Remove and dispose of gloves. *Comments:*	☐	☐	☐	
7. Wash your hands. *Comments:*	☐	☐	☐	
8. Place call signal within easy reach of the patient and provide privacy, if possible. *Comments:*	☐	☐	☐	
9. Watch for the patient's signal and answer his call immediately. *Comments:*	☐	☐	☐	
10. Wash your hands. *Comments:*	☐	☐	☐	
11. Fill the basin with warm water and place it next to the soap, washcloth, and towel on the overbed table so the patient may wash his hands. *Comments:*	☐	☐	☐	

continued on the following page

continued from the previous page

Procedure 76	Able to Perform	Able to Perform with Assistance	Unable to Perform	Initials and Date
12. Apply disposable gloves. *Comments:*	☐	☐	☐	
13. Ask the patient to hand you the urinal. *Comments:*	☐	☐	☐	
14. Cover the urinal. *Comments:*	☐	☐	☐	
15. Rearrange the bedclothes. *Comments:*	☐	☐	☐	
16. Take the urinal to the bathroom or utility room and observe contents. *Comments:*	☐	☐	☐	
17. Measure contents if required. *Comments:*	☐	☐	☐	
18. Empty unless you observe anything unusual. If so, save the contents for the nurse to inspect. *Comments:*	☐	☐	☐	
19. Turn on the faucet using a paper towel. *Comments:*	☐	☐	☐	
20. Rinse the urinal with cold water and clean it with warm, soapy water. *Comments:*	☐	☐	☐	
21. Rinse, dry, and cover the urinal. *Comments:*	☐	☐	☐	
22. Remove and dispose of gloves. *Comments:*	☐	☐	☐	
23. Wash your hands. *Comments:*	☐	☐	☐	
24. Place the urinal inside the patient's bedside table. *Comments:*	☐	☐	☐	
25. Clean and replace other articles. *Comments:*	☐	☐	☐	
26. Carry out procedure completion actions. *Comments:*	☐	☐	☐	

Checklist for Procedure 77 Assisting with Use of the Bedside Commode

Name _____ Date _____

School _____

Instructor _____

Course _____

Procedure 77 Assisting with Use of the Bedside Commode	Able to Perform	Able to Perform with Assistance	Unable to Perform	Initials and Date
1. Carry out beginning procedure actions. *Comments:*	☐	☐	☐	
2. Assemble equipment. *Comments:*	☐	☐	☐	
3. Position the commode beside the bed, facing the head. *Comments:*	☐	☐	☐	
4. Lock the commode wheels and open the lid. *Comments:*	☐	☐	☐	
5. Check to be sure the receptacle is under the seat. *Comments:*	☐	☐	☐	
6. Lower the side rail nearest you, lower the bed to the lowest horizontal position, and lock the bed wheels. *Comments:*	☐	☐	☐	
7. Apply disposable gloves. *Comments:*	☐	☐	☐	
8. Assist the patient to a sitting position. *Comments:*	☐	☐	☐	
9. Swing the patient's legs over the edge of the bed. *Comments:*	☐	☐	☐	
10. Assist the patient to put on a robe and slippers. *Comments:*	☐	☐	☐	
11. Assist the patient to stand. Apply a transfer belt if necessary. *Comments:*	☐	☐	☐	

continued on the following page

continued from the previous page

Procedure 77	Able to Perform	Able to Perform with Assistance	Unable to Perform	Initials and Date
12. Support the patient with hands on either side of the chest. *Comments:*	☐	☐	☐	
13. Pivot the patient to the right and lower her to the commode. *Comments:*	☐	☐	☐	
14. Cover the patient's legs with a bath blanket. *Comments:*	☐	☐	☐	
15. Leave the call signal and tissue within easy reach. *Comments:*	☐	☐	☐	
16. Remove and discard gloves. *Comments:*	☐	☐	☐	
17. Watch for the patient's signal and answer her call immediately. *Comments:*	☐	☐	☐	
18. Wash your hands and apply disposable gloves. *Comments:*	☐	☐	☐	
19. Fill a basin with water at 105°F and take it to the bedside table along with soap, a towel, and a washcloth. *Comments:*	☐	☐	☐	
20. Remove the bath blanket and assist the patient to stand. *Comments:*	☐	☐	☐	
21. Cleanse the anus and perineum if the patient is unable to do so. *Comments:*	☐	☐	☐	
22. Allow the patient to wash and dry her hands. *Comments:*	☐	☐	☐	
23. Remove and dispose of gloves. *Comments:*	☐	☐	☐	

Procedure 77	Able to Perform	Able to Perform with Assistance	Unable to Perform	Initials and Date
24. Wash your hands. *Comments:*	☐	☐	☐	
25. Assist the patient to return to bed and adjust the bedding and pillows for comfort. *Comments:*	☐	☐	☐	
26. Leave the call signal within easy reach. *Comments:*	☐	☐	☐	
27. Apply disposable gloves. *Comments:*	☐	☐	☐	
28. Remove and cover the receptacle from the commode and close the lid. *Comments:*	☐	☐	☐	
29. Take the receptacle to the bathroom and note its content. Measure if required. *Comments:*	☐	☐	☐	
30. Empty and clean the receptacle. *Comments:*	☐	☐	☐	
31. Replace the receptacle in the commode. *Comments:*	☐	☐	☐	
32. Remove and dispose of gloves. *Comments:*	☐	☐	☐	
33. Properly store the commode. *Comments:*	☐	☐	☐	
34. Carry out procedure completion actions. *Comments:*	☐	☐	☐	
35. Empty unless you observe anything unusual. If so, save the contents for the nurse to inspect. *Comments:*	☐	☐	☐	

Checklist for Procedure 78   Assisting the Patient Who Can Feed Self

Name _____ Date _____

School _____

Instructor _____

Course _____

Procedure 78 Assisting the Patient Who Can Feed Self	Able to Perform	Able to Perform with Assistance	Unable to Perform	Initials and Date
1. Carry out beginning procedure actions. *Comments:*	☐	☐	☐	
2. Assemble equipment. *Comments:*	☐	☐	☐	
3. Offer bedpan/urinal and if needed apply gloves. *Comments:*	☐	☐	☐	
4. Elevate the head of the bed or assist the patient out of bed, if permitted. *Comments:*	☐	☐	☐	
5. Provide a washcloth for the patient to use. *Comments:*	☐	☐	☐	
6. Assist with oral hygiene or dentures. *Comments:*	☐	☐	☐	
7. Remove and discard gloves. *Comments:*	☐	☐	☐	
8. Clear off the overbed table. *Comments:*	☐	☐	☐	
9. Position the table in front of the patient. *Comments:*	☐	☐	☐	
10. Wash your hands. *Comments:*	☐	☐	☐	
11. Obtain the meal tray. *Comments:*	☐	☐	☐	

continued on the following page

continued from the previous page

Procedure 78	Able to Perform	Able to Perform with Assistance	Unable to Perform	Initials and Date
12. Check the diet with the dietary card and with the patient's identification band. *Comments:*	☐	☐	☐	
13. Place the tray on the overbed table. *Comments:*	☐	☐	☐	
14. Arrange the food in a convenient manner. *Comments:*	☐	☐	☐	
15. Assist the patient as needed. *Comments:*	☐	☐	☐	
16. Remove the tray as soon as the patient is finished. *Comments:*	☐	☐	☐	
17. Note what the patient has eaten and not eaten. *Comments:*	☐	☐	☐	
18. Record fluid and food intake. *Comments:*	☐	☐	☐	
19. Push the overbed table out of the way. *Comments:*	☐	☐	☐	
20. Carry out procedure completion actions. *Comments:*	☐	☐	☐	

Checklist for Procedure 79   Feeding the Dependent Patient

Name _____ Date _____

School _____

Instructor _____

Course _____

Procedure 79 Feeding the Dependent Patient	Able to Perform	Able to Perform with Assistance	Unable to Perform	Initials and Date
1. Carry out beginning procedure actions. Comments:	☐	☐	☐	
2. Assemble equipment. Comments:	☐	☐	☐	
3. Offer bedpan/urinal and if needed apply gloves. Comments:	☐	☐	☐	
4. Provide oral hygiene. Comments:	☐	☐	☐	
5. Clear off the overbed table. Comments:	☐	☐	☐	
6. Elevate the head of the bed with the patient's head bent slightly forward. Comments:	☐	☐	☐	
7. Place a towel or protector under the patient's chin. Comments:	☐	☐	☐	
8. Obtain the meal tray. Comments:	☐	☐	☐	
9. Check the diet with the dietary card and with the patient's identification band. Comments:	☐	☐	☐	
10. Place the tray on the overbed table. Comments:	☐	☐	☐	

continued on the following page

continued from the previous page

Procedure 79	Able to Perform	Able to Perform with Assistance	Unable to Perform	Initials and Date
11. Butter bread and cut meat. *Comments:*	☐	☐	☐	
12. Use different drinking straws for each liquid. *Comments:*	☐	☐	☐	
13. Use adaptive devices as indicated. *Comments:*	☐	☐	☐	
14. Sit at eye level with the patient. *Comments:*	☐	☐	☐	
15. Hold the spoon at a right angle. *Comments:*	☐	☐	☐	
16. Give solid foods from the point of the spoon. *Comments:*	☐	☐	☐	
17. Alternate solids and liquids. *Comments:*	☐	☐	☐	
18. Describe or show the patient what kind of food she has and ask in what order she would like it served. *Comments:*	☐	☐	☐	
19. Direct food to the unaffected side of a stroke patient. *Comments:*	☐	☐	☐	
20. Check for food stored in the affected side of a stroke patient. *Comments:*	☐	☐	☐	
21. Watch patient's throat for swallowing. *Comments:*	☐	☐	☐	
22. Test hot foods before feeding them to the patient. *Comments:*	☐	☐	☐	
23. Never blow on or taste the patient's food. *Comments:*	☐	☐	☐	

Procedure 79	Able to Perform	Able to Perform with Assistance	Unable to Perform	Initials and Date
24. Do not hurry the meal. *Comments:*	☐	☐	☐	
25. Allow the patient to assist if able. *Comments:*	☐	☐	☐	
26. Wipe the patient's mouth as necessary. *Comments:*	☐	☐	☐	
27. Remove the tray as soon as the patient is finished. *Comments:*	☐	☐	☐	
28. Record fluid and food intake. *Comments:*	☐	☐	☐	
29. Carry out procedure completion actions. *Comments:*	☐	☐	☐	

Checklist for Procedure 80   Applying an Ice Bag

Name _____ Date _____

School _____

Instructor _____

Course _____

Procedure 80 Applying an Ice Bag	Able to Perform	Able to Perform with Assistance	Unable to Perform	Initials and Date
1. Assemble equipment. *Comments:*	☐	☐	☐	
2. Fill the ice bag with water and check for leaks. *Comments:*	☐	☐	☐	
3. Empty the bag. *Comments:*	☐	☐	☐	
4. Rinse ice cubes in water to remove sharp edges. Use crushed ice if possible. *Comments:*	☐	☐	☐	
5. Fill the ice bag half full of ice. *Comments:*	☐	☐	☐	
6. Rest the ice bag on a flat surface, place top on loosely, and press to remove air from the bag. *Comments:*	☐	☐	☐	
7. Fasten the top securely. *Comments:*	☐	☐	☐	
8. Test for leakage. *Comments:*	☐	☐	☐	
9. Wipe the ice bag dry with paper towels and place in a cloth cover. *Comments:*	☐	☐	☐	
10. Take equipment to the bedside on a tray. *Comments:*	☐	☐	☐	

continued on the following page

continued from the previous page

Procedure 80	Able to Perform	Able to Perform with Assistance	Unable to Perform	Initials and Date
11. Carry out beginning procedure actions. *Comments:*	☐	☐	☐	
12. Apply the ice bag to the affected area. *Comments:*	☐	☐	☐	
13. Refill the ice bag before all of the ice has melted. *Comments:*	☐	☐	☐	
14. Check the skin under the ice bag every 10 minutes. *Comments:*	☐	☐	☐	
15. Continue the cold application for the specified time. *Comments:*	☐	☐	☐	
16. Carry out procedure completion actions. *Comments:*	☐	☐	☐	
17. When treatment is complete, wash the bag with soap and water. *Comments:*	☐	☐	☐	
18. Rinse and dry completely; then screw top on. *Comments:*	☐	☐	☐	
19. Wipe the bag with disinfectant according to policy. *Comments:*	☐	☐	☐	
20. Leave air in the bag. *Comments:*	☐	☐	☐	
21. Wash reusable cold pack with soap and water or wipe with disinfectant. *Comments:*	☐	☐	☐	
22. Return the pack to the refrigerator. *Comments:*	☐	☐	☐	

Checklist for Procedure 81   Applying a Disposable Cold Pack

Name _____ Date _____

School _____

Instructor _____

Course _____

Procedure 81 Applying a Disposable Cold Pack	Able to Perform	Able to Perform with Assistance	Unable to Perform	Initials and Date
1. Carry out beginning procedure actions. *Comments:*	☐	☐	☐	
2. Assemble equipment. *Comments:*	☐	☐	☐	
3. Expose the area to be treated. *Comments:*	☐	☐	☐	
4. Place the cold pack in a cloth covering. *Comments:*	☐	☐	☐	
5. Activate the cold pack chemicals. *Comments:*	☐	☐	☐	
6. Place the covered cold pack on the proper area and cover with a towel. *Comments:*	☐	☐	☐	
7. Note the time of application. *Comments:*	☐	☐	☐	
8. Secure the cover with tape or gauze, if necessary. *Comments:*	☐	☐	☐	
9. Leave the patient in a comfortable position. *Comments:*	☐	☐	☐	
10. Place the call signal within easy reach. *Comments:*	☐	☐	☐	
11. Return to the bedside every 10 minutes. *Comments:*	☐	☐	☐	

continued on the following page

continued from the previous page

Procedure 81	Able to Perform	Able to Perform with Assistance	Unable to Perform	Initials and Date
12. Check the area for discoloration or numbness. *Comments:*	☐	☐	☐	
13. Remove the pack after 30 minutes or after the specified treatment time. *Comments:*	☐	☐	☐	
14. Remove the pack from the cover and discard. *Comments:*	☐	☐	☐	
15. Put the cover in a laundry hamper. *Comments:*	☐	☐	☐	
16. Carry out procedure completion actions. *Comments:*	☐	☐	☐	

Checklist for Procedure 82   Applying an Aquamatic K-Pad®

Name _____ Date _____

School _____

Instructor _____

Course _____

Procedure 82 Applying an Aquamatic K-Pad®	Able to Perform	Able to Perform with Assistance	Unable to Perform	Initials and Date
1. Carry out beginning procedure actions. *Comments:*	☐	☐	☐	
2. Assemble equipment. *Comments:*	☐	☐	☐	
3. Check the unit to ensure it is in working order. *Comments:*	☐	☐	☐	
4. Place the control unit on the bedside table. *Comments:*	☐	☐	☐	
5. Check the level of the distilled water; if low fill two-thirds full or to fill line. *Comments:*	☐	☐	☐	
6. Clear the tubing of air. *Comments:*	☐	☐	☐	
7. Screw the cover in place and loosen it one-quarter turn. *Comments:*	☐	☐	☐	
8. Select the proper temperature before turning the unit on. *Comments:*	☐	☐	☐	
9. Plug in the unit. *Comments:*	☐	☐	☐	
10. Cover the pad with an appropriate cover. *Comments:*	☐	☐	☐	
11. Expose the area to be treated. *Comments:*	☐	☐	☐	

continued on the following page

continued from the previous page

Procedure 82	Able to Perform	Able to Perform with Assistance	Unable to Perform	Initials and Date
12. Place the covered pad on the patient and note the time. *Comments:*	☐	☐	☐	
13. Coil the tubing on the bed to promote fluid flow. *Comments:*	☐	☐	☐	
14. Periodically check the skin under the pad. *Comments:*	☐	☐	☐	
15. Check the level of the water in the control unit and refill if necessary. *Comments:*	☐	☐	☐	
16. Remove the pad after specified treatment time. *Comments:*	☐	☐	☐	
17. Carry out procedure completion actions. *Comments:*	☐	☐	☐	

Checklist for Procedure 83   Performing a Warm Soak

Name _____ Date _____

School _____

Instructor _____

Course _____

Procedure 83 Performing a Warm Soak	Able to Perform	Able to Perform with Assistance	Unable to Perform	Initials and Date
1. Carry out beginning procedure actions. *Comments:*	☐	☐	☐	
2. Assemble equipment. *Comments:*	☐	☐	☐	
3. Take equipment to the bedside. *Comments:*	☐	☐	☐	
4. Cover the patient with a bath blanket. *Comments:*	☐	☐	☐	
5. Fanfold bedding to the foot of the bed. *Comments:*	☐	☐	☐	
6. Expose the limb to be soaked. *Comments:*	☐	☐	☐	
7. Raise and secure the side rail. *Comments:*	☐	☐	☐	
8. Position the patient for comfort on the far side of the bed. *Comments:*	☐	☐	☐	
9. Cover the bed with a plastic sheet or towel. *Comments:*	☐	☐	☐	
10. Fill a soak basin with warm water. *Comments:*	☐	☐	☐	
11. Check to ensure prescribed temperature with a bath thermometer. *Comments:*	☐	☐	☐	
12. Position the soak basin on the bed protector. *Comments:*	☐	☐	☐	

continued on the following page

continued from the previous page

Procedure 83	Able to Perform	Able to Perform with Assistance	Unable to Perform	Initials and Date
13. Assist the patient to gradually place limb in basin. *Comments:*	☐	☐	☐	
14. Cover the basin with a towel. *Comments:*	☐	☐	☐	
15. Check the temperature every 5 minutes. *Comments:*	☐	☐	☐	
16. Remove limb and add warm water to the soak basin if necessary to maintain correct temperature. *Comments:*	☐	☐	☐	
17. After soaking for the prescribed time, lift the patient's limb out of the basin. *Comments:*	☐	☐	☐	
18. Slip the basin forward and allow the limb to rest on the bath towel. *Comments:*	☐	☐	☐	
19. Place the basin on the overbed table. *Comments:*	☐	☐	☐	
20. Gently pat the limb dry with a towel. *Comments:*	☐	☐	☐	
21. Remove the plastic sheet and towel. *Comments:*	☐	☐	☐	
22. Adjust bedding and remove the bath blanket. *Comments:*	☐	☐	☐	
23. Fold and store the bath blanket for reuse if necessary. *Comments:*	☐	☐	☐	
24. Place the call signal within the patient's reach. *Comments:*	☐	☐	☐	
25. Lower the head of the bed and make the patient comfortable. *Comments:*	☐	☐	☐	
26. Take the equipment to the utility room; clean and store according to policy. *Comments:*	☐	☐	☐	
27. Carry out procedure completion actions. *Comments:*	☐	☐	☐	

Checklist for Procedure 84   Applying a Warm Moist Compress

Name _____ Date _____

School _____

Instructor _____

Course _____

Procedure 84 Applying a Warm Moist Compress	Able to Perform	Able to Perform with Assistance	Unable to Perform	Initials and Date
1. Carry out beginning procedure actions. *Comments:*	☐	☐	☐	
2. Assemble equipment. *Comments:*	☐	☐	☐	
3. Take equipment to the bedside. *Comments:*	☐	☐	☐	
4. Expose only the area to be treated. *Comments:*	☐	☐	☐	
5. Cover the bed with a towel. *Comments:*	☐	☐	☐	
6. Apply disposable gloves. *Comments:*	☐	☐	☐	
7. Check the temperature of the solution. *Comments:*	☐	☐	☐	
8. Moisten the compress and remove excess water. *Comments:*	☐	☐	☐	
9. Apply to the treatment area. *Comments:*	☐	☐	☐	
10. Secure the compress. *Comments:*	☐	☐	☐	
11. Help the patient to maintain a comfortable position during treatment. *Comments:*	☐	☐	☐	

continued on the following page

continued from the previous page

Procedure 84	Able to Perform	Able to Perform with Assistance	Unable to Perform	Initials and Date
12. Unscreen the unit and place the call signal within the patient's reach. *Comments:*	☐	☐	☐	
13. Maintain proper temperature and moisture. *Comments:*	☐	☐	☐	
14. Remove the compress when ordered. *Comments:*	☐	☐	☐	
15. Change the compress as ordered or once in 24 hours. *Comments:*	☐	☐	☐	
16. Check the patient's skin several times each day. *Comments:*	☐	☐	☐	
17. Discard the compress when treatment is complete. *Comments:*	☐	☐	☐	
18. Remove and dispose of gloves. *Comments:*	☐	☐	☐	
19. Carry out procedure completion actions. *Comments:*	☐	☐	☐	

Checklist for Procedure 85   Assisting with Application of a Hypothermia Blanket

Name _____ Date _____

School _____

Instructor _____

Course _____

Procedure 85 Assisting with Application of a Hypothermia Blanket	Able to Perform	Able to Perform with Assistance	Unable to Perform	Initials and Date
1. Wash your hands. *Comments:*	☐	☐	☐	
2. Collect equipment and take to the bedside. *Comments:*	☐	☐	☐	
3. Assemble equipment. *Comments:*	☐	☐	☐	
4. Set up equipment, check for safety, and check that control unit is grounded. *Comments:*	☐	☐	☐	
5. Connect the blanket to the control unit and set the control. *Comments:*	☐	☐	☐	
6. Turn unit on and add liquid. *Comments:*	☐	☐	☐	
7. Prepare the patient as the blanket precools. *Comments:*	☐	☐	☐	
8. Carry out beginning procedure actions. *Comments:*	☐	☐	☐	
9. Place a hospital-type gown on the patient. *Comments:*	☐	☐	☐	
10. Measure and record vital signs. *Comments:*	☐	☐	☐	
11. Place the blanket on the bed and cover with a sheet. *Comments:*	☐	☐	☐	

continued on the following page

continued from the previous page

Procedure 85	Able to Perform	Able to Perform with Assistance	Unable to Perform	Initials and Date
12. Position the patient in a recumbent position on the thermal blanket. *Comments:*	☐	☐	☐	
13. Place a pillow under the patient's head, but not touching the blanket. *Comments:*	☐	☐	☐	
14. Wash your hands. *Comments:*	☐	☐	☐	
15. Apply disposable gloves. *Comments:*	☐	☐	☐	
16. Insert a rectal thermometer into the patient's rectum and tape in place. *Comments:*	☐	☐	☐	
17. Plug the end of the probe into the proper jack on the control panel. *Comments:*	☐	☐	☐	
18. Place a second sheet over the patient and place a second thermal blanket over the sheet, if ordered. *Comments:*	☐	☐	☐	
19. Apply lanolin-based cream to the patient's skin where it contacts the blanket. *Comments:*	☐	☐	☐	
20. Remove and discard gloves. *Comments:*	☐	☐	☐	
21. Wash your hands. *Comments:*	☐	☐	☐	
22. Monitor vital signs, neurological response, and intake and output every 5 minutes. *Comments:*	☐	☐	☐	
23. When desired temperature is reached, monitor every 15 minutes or as ordered. *Comments:*	☐	☐	☐	

Procedure 85	Able to Perform	Able to Perform with Assistance	Unable to Perform	Initials and Date
24. Report color changes or excessive shivering. *Comments:*	☐	☐	☐	
25. Reposition the patient every 30 minutes to 1 hour. *Comments:*	☐	☐	☐	
26. Reapply skin cream and change gown as necessary. *Comments:*	☐	☐	☐	
27. At completion of treatment, turn off the unit. *Comments:*	☐	☐	☐	
28. Disconnect the blanket(s) and return them to storage. *Comments:*	☐	☐	☐	
29. Apply disposable gloves. *Comments:*	☐	☐	☐	
30. Continue to monitor the patient as you remove equipment. *Comments:*	☐	☐	☐	
31. Replace any damp bedding or garments and cover the patient. *Comments:*	☐	☐	☐	
32. Continue to monitor the patient every 30 minutes until stable. *Comments:*	☐	☐	☐	
33. Clean thermometer probe and store. *Comments:*	☐	☐	☐	
34. Remove and discard gloves. *Comments:*	☐	☐	☐	
35. Carry out procedure completion actions. *Comments:*	☐	☐	☐	

Checklist for Procedure 86   Assisting with a Physical Examination

Name _____ Date _____

School _____

Instructor _____

Course _____

Procedure 86 **Assisting with a Physical Examination**	Able to Perform	Able to Perform with Assistance	Unable to Perform	Initials and Date
1. Carry out beginning procedure actions. *Comments:*	☐	☐	☐	
2. Assemble equipment. *Comments:*	☐	☐	☐	
3. If ambulatory, have the patient use the restroom; if nonambulatory, offer a bedpan or urinal. *Comments:*	☐	☐	☐	
4. Help the patient onto the examination table. *Comments:*	☐	☐	☐	
5. Cover the patient with a drape. *Comments:*	☐	☐	☐	
6. Provide privacy. *Comments:*	☐	☐	☐	
7. Position the patient and equipment as necessary. *Comments:*	☐	☐	☐	
8. Hand equipment to the examiner. *Comments:*	☐	☐	☐	
9. Adjust lighting as necessary. *Comments:*	☐	☐	☐	
10. After the examination, help the patient to sit up slowly, get off the table, stand, dress, and return to the unit or office. *Comments:*	☐	☐	☐	

continued on the following page

continued from the previous page

Procedure 86	Able to Perform	Able to Perform with Assistance	Unable to Perform	Initials and Date
11. Wash your hands. *Comments:*	☐	☐	☐	
12. Return to the examination room and apply gloves. *Comments:*	☐	☐	☐	
13. Clean equipment. *Comments:*	☐	☐	☐	
14. Care for specimens according to policy. *Comments:*	☐	☐	☐	
15. Remove and dispose of gloves. *Comments:*	☐	☐	☐	
16. Wash your hands. *Comments:*	☐	☐	☐	
17. Carry out procedure completion actions. *Comments:*	☐	☐	☐	

Checklist for Procedure 87   Shaving the Operative Area

Name _____   Date _____

School _____

Instructor _____

Course _____

Procedure 87 **Shaving the Operative Area**	Able to Perform	Able to Perform with Assistance	Unable to Perform	Initials and Date
1. Carry out beginning procedure actions. *Comments:*	☐	☐	☐	
2. Assemble equipment. *Comments:*	☐	☐	☐	
3. Determine the exact area to be prepped. *Comments:*	☐	☐	☐	
4. Fill two small bowls with warm water and add cleansing soap to one. *Comments:*	☐	☐	☐	
5. Adjust the razor and blade and make sure both are tight. *Comments:*	☐	☐	☐	
6. Cover the tray and carry to the bedside. *Comments:*	☐	☐	☐	
7. Drape the patient with a bath blanket. *Comments:*	☐	☐	☐	
8. Place a towel or protector under the area to be shaved. *Comments:*	☐	☐	☐	
9. Apply disposable gloves. *Comments:*	☐	☐	☐	
10. Clip the hair if necessary. *Comments:*	☐	☐	☐	
11. Soften the hairs if using a safety razor and blade with a soapy solution. *Comments:*	☐	☐	☐	
12. Hold the skin taut with one hand and lather the area to be shaved. *Comments:*	☐	☐	☐	

continued on the following page

continued from the previous page

Procedure 87	Able to Perform	Able to Perform with Assistance	Unable to Perform	Initials and Date
13. Hold the razor at a 45-degree angle. *Comments:*	☐	☐	☐	
14. Shave the area with strokes in the same direction as hair growth. *Comments:*	☐	☐	☐	
15. Work carefully around warts and moles. *Comments:*	☐	☐	☐	
16. Using applicators, clean umbilicus area and shave if it is in the operative area. *Comments:*	☐	☐	☐	
17. Check carefully for hairs after shaving and remove gently if found. *Comments:*	☐	☐	☐	
18. Cleanse skin with warm, soapy water. *Comments:*	☐	☐	☐	
19. Rinse and dry thoroughly. *Comments:*	☐	☐	☐	
20. Dispose of equipment. *Comments:*	☐	☐	☐	
21. Remove the towel from under the patient. *Comments:*	☐	☐	☐	
22. Raise side rails. *Comments:*	☐	☐	☐	
23. Change linen if necessary. *Comments:*	☐	☐	☐	
24. Remove and dispose of gloves. *Comments:*	☐	☐	☐	
25. Carry out procedure completion actions. *Comments:*	☐	☐	☐	

Checklist for Procedure 88   Assisting the Patient to Deep Breathe and Cough

Name _____ Date _____

School _____

Instructor _____

Course _____

Procedure 88 Assisting the Patient to Deep Breathe and Cough	Able to Perform	Able to Perform with Assistance	Unable to Perform	Initials and Date
1. Carry out beginning procedure actions. *Comments:*	☐	☐	☐	
2. Assemble equipment. *Comments:*	☐	☐	☐	
3. Elevate the head of the bed. *Comments:*	☐	☐	☐	
4. Assist the patient into a semi-Fowler's position. *Comments:*	☐	☐	☐	
5. Instruct the patient to place his hands on either side of his rib cage or over the operative site. *Comments:*	☐	☐	☐	
6. Ask the patient to take as a deep breath as possible and hold for 3 to 5 seconds. *Comments:*	☐	☐	☐	
7. Have the patient exhale slowly through pursed lips. *Comments:*	☐	☐	☐	
8. Repeat this exercise about five times unless the patient seems too tired. *Comments:*	☐	☐	☐	
9. If the patient seems too tired, stop the procedure and report to nurse. *Comments:*	☐	☐	☐	
10. Place a pillow over the incision line. *Comments:*	☐	☐	☐	

continued on the following page

continued from the previous page

Procedure 88	Able to Perform	Able to Perform with Assistance	Unable to Perform	Initials and Date
11. Have the patient hold the pillow on either side or interlace fingers across incision to act as a brace. *Comments:*	☐	☐	☐	
12. Give tissues to the patient. *Comments:*	☐	☐	☐	
13. Instruct the patient to take a deep breath and cough forcefully twice with the mouth open. *Comments:*	☐	☐	☐	
14. Collect any secretions that are brought up in the tissues. *Comments:*	☐	☐	☐	
15. Apply disposable gloves. *Comments:*	☐	☐	☐	
16. Dispose of tissues in emesis basin. *Comments:*	☐	☐	☐	
17. Assist the patient to a new comfortable position. *Comments:*	☐	☐	☐	
18. Clean the emesis basin. *Comments:*	☐	☐	☐	
19. Remove and dispose of gloves. *Comments:*	☐	☐	☐	
20. Carry out procedure completion actions. *Comments:*	☐	☐	☐	
21. Report observations to the nurse. *Comments:*	☐	☐	☐	

Checklist for Procedure 89   Performing Postoperative Leg Exercises

Name _____ Date _____

School _____

Instructor _____

Course _____

Procedure 89 Performing Postoperative Leg Exercises	Able to Perform	Able to Perform with Assistance	Unable to Perform	Initials and Date
1. Carry out beginning procedure actions. *Comments:*	☐	☐	☐	
2. Explain the procedure to the patient. *Comments:*	☐	☐	☐	
3. Lower the side rail. *Comments:*	☐	☐	☐	
4. Cover the patient with a bath blanket. *Comments:*	☐	☐	☐	
5. Draw the top bedding to the foot of the bed. *Comments:*	☐	☐	☐	
6. Supervise exercises or assist as needed. *Comments:*	☐	☐	☐	
7. Have the patient brace the incisional area with laced hands. *Comments:*	☐	☐	☐	
8. Instruct the patient to rotate each ankle by drawing imaginary circles with her toes. *Comments:*	☐	☐	☐	
9. Have the patient dorsiflex and plantar flex each ankle. *Comments:*	☐	☐	☐	
10. Have the patient flex and extend each knee and each hip. *Comments:*	☐	☐	☐	

continued on the following page

continued from the previous page

Procedure 89	Able to Perform	Able to Perform with Assistance	Unable to Perform	Initials and Date
11. Repeat each exercise three to five times, assisting as necessary. *Comments:*	☐	☐	☐	
12. Apply or reapply support hose as ordered after exercises. *Comments:*	☐	☐	☐	
13. Draw bedding up and remove bath blanket. *Comments:*	☐	☐	☐	
14. Fold the bath blanket and place in the bedside stand for reuse. *Comments:*	☐	☐	☐	
15. Carry out procedure completion actions. *Comments:*	☐	☐	☐	
16. Report the outcome of the exercises to the nurse. *Comments:*	☐	☐	☐	

Checklist for Procedure 90   Applying Elasticized Stockings

Name _____ Date _____

School _____

Instructor _____

Course _____

Procedure 90 Applying Elasticized Stockings	Able to Perform	Able to Perform with Assistance	Unable to Perform	Initials and Date
1. Carry out beginning procedure actions. *Comments:*	☐	☐	☐	
2. Assemble equipment. *Comments:*	☐	☐	☐	
3. Instruct the patient to lie down. *Comments:*	☐	☐	☐	
4. Expose the patient's legs one at a time. *Comments:*	☐	☐	☐	
5. Grasp the stocking with both hands at the top and roll it toward the toe end. *Comments:*	☐	☐	☐	
6. Adjust over the patient's toes, positioning the opening at the base of the toes. *Comments:*	☐	☐	☐	
7. Apply the stocking to the leg by rolling it upward toward the body. *Comments:*	☐	☐	☐	
8. Check to be sure that the stocking is applied evenly and smoothly with no wrinkles. *Comments:*	☐	☐	☐	
9. Repeat procedure for the opposite leg. *Comments:*	☐	☐	☐	
10. Carry out procedure completion actions. *Comments:*	☐	☐	☐	

Checklist for Procedure 91 Applying Elastic Bandage

Name _____ Date _____

School _____

Instructor _____

Course _____

Procedure 91 Applying Elastic Bandage	Able to Perform	Able to Perform with Assistance	Unable to Perform	Initials and Date
1. Carry out beginning procedure actions. *Comments:*	☐	☐	☐	
2. Assemble equipment. *Comments:*	☐	☐	☐	
3. Check the area to be bandaged. *Comments:*	☐	☐	☐	
4. Elevate the arm or leg for 15 to 30 minutes before application. *Comments:*	☐	☐	☐	
5. Apply the bandage so two skin surfaces do not rub together. *Comments:*	☐	☐	☐	
6. Pad areas with gauze or cotton to prevent friction. *Comments:*	☐	☐	☐	
7. Hold the bandage with the roll facing upward in one hand and the free end of the bandage in your other hand. *Comments:*	☐	☐	☐	
8. Hold the roll close to the part being bandaged so the pressure is even. *Comments:*	☐	☐	☐	
9. Always wrap an extremity from distal area to proximal area. *Comments:*	☐	☐	☐	
10. Unroll the bandage as you wrap the body part. *Comments:*	☐	☐	☐	

continued on the following page

continued from the previous page

Procedure 91	Able to Perform	Able to Perform with Assistance	Unable to Perform	Initials and Date
11. Overlap each layer of bandage by one-half the width of the strip. Ensure it is smooth and wrinkle free. *Comments:*	☐	☐	☐	
12. Secure the bandage with pins, tape, or self-closures. *Comments:*	☐	☐	☐	
13. Check distal circulation just after application and once or twice every 8 hours thereafter. *Comments:*	☐	☐	☐	
14. Remove and reapply the bandage every shift, or more often if needed. *Comments:*	☐	☐	☐	
15. Check with the nurse to see if bandage should be worn continuously or only at specified times. *Comments:*	☐	☐	☐	
16. Carry out procedure completion actions. *Comments:*	☐	☐	☐	

Checklist for Procedure 92   Applying Pneumatic Compression Hosiery

Name _____ Date _____

School _____

Instructor _____

Course _____

Procedure 92 **Applying Pneumatic Compression Hosiery**	Able to Perform	Able to Perform with Assistance	Unable to Perform	Initials and Date
1. Carry out beginning procedure actions. *Comments:*	☐	☐	☐	
2. Assemble equipment. *Comments:*	☐	☐	☐	
3. Open the hose and lay them flat on the bed with markings opposite the knee and ankle. *Comments:*	☐	☐	☐	
4. Lift the patient's leg and slide the hose under it. *Comments:*	☐	☐	☐	
5. Begin on the side opposite the plastic tubing. *Comments:*	☐	☐	☐	
6. Wrap the sleeve smoothly around the leg with the opening in front, over the knee. *Comments:*	☐	☐	☐	
7. Beginning at the ankle, fasten the Velcro fasteners securely. *Comments:*	☐	☐	☐	
8. Secure the ankle and calf, then the thigh. *Comments:*	☐	☐	☐	
9. Insert two fingers between the sleeve and the patient's leg to check the fit. *Comments:*	☐	☐	☐	
10. Wrap the other leg in the same manner. *Comments:*	☐	☐	☐	

continued on the following page

continued from the previous page

Procedure 92	Able to Perform	Able to Perform with Assistance	Unable to Perform	Initials and Date
11. Attach the plastic tubing on each leg to the compression controller. *Comments:*	☐	☐	☐	
12. Plug in the controller and turn on the power. *Comments:*	☐	☐	☐	
13. Remain with the patient for one complete cycle. *Comments:*	☐	☐	☐	
14. Carry out procedure completion actions. *Comments:*	☐	☐	☐	

Checklist for Procedure 93 Assisting the Patient to Dangle

Name _____ Date _____

School _____

Instructor _____

Course _____

Procedure 93 Assisting the Patient to Dangle	Able to Perform	Able to Perform with Assistance	Unable to Perform	Initials and Date
1. Carry out beginning procedure actions. *Comments:*	☐	☐	☐	
2. Assemble equipment. *Comments:*	☐	☐	☐	
3. Check the patient's pulse. *Comments:*	☐	☐	☐	
4. Lower the side rail nearest you. *Comments:*	☐	☐	☐	
5. Lock the bed at the lowest position. *Comments:*	☐	☐	☐	
6. Drape the patient with a bath blanket. *Comments:*	☐	☐	☐	
7. Fanfold top cover to the foot of the bed. *Comments:*	☐	☐	☐	
8. Gradually elevate the head of the bed. *Comments:*	☐	☐	☐	
9. Help the patient to put on a bathrobe. *Comments:*	☐	☐	☐	
10. Place one arm around the patient's shoulders and the other arm under the knees. *Comments:*	☐	☐	☐	
11. Gently and slowly turn the patient toward you. *Comments:*	☐	☐	☐	

continued on the following page

continued from the previous page

Procedure 93	Able to Perform	Able to Perform with Assistance	Unable to Perform	Initials and Date
12. Allow the patient's legs to hang over the side of the bed. *Comments:*	☐	☐	☐	
13. Roll a pillow and tuck it firmly against the patient's back. *Comments:*	☐	☐	☐	
14. Put on the patient's slippers and ask him to swing his legs. *Comments:*	☐	☐	☐	
15. Have the patient dangle as long as ordered. *Comments:*	☐	☐	☐	
16. Check the patient's pulse. *Comments:*	☐	☐	☐	
17. Rearrange the pillow at the head of the bed. *Comments:*	☐	☐	☐	
18. Remove the patient's bathrobe and slippers. *Comments:*	☐	☐	☐	
19. Place one arm around the patient's shoulders and the other arm under the knees. *Comments:*	☐	☐	☐	
20. Gently and slowly swing the patient's legs onto the bed. *Comments:*	☐	☐	☐	
21. Check the patient's pulse. *Comments:*	☐	☐	☐	
22. Lower the head of the bed and raise the side rails. *Comments:*	☐	☐	☐	
23. Carry out procedure completion actions. *Comments:*	☐	☐	☐	
24. Wash your hands. *Comments:*	☐	☐	☐	
25. Report completion of your task to the nurse. *Comments:*	☐	☐	☐	

Checklist for Procedure 94   Giving Postmortem Care

Name _____ Date _____

School _____

Instructor _____

Course _____

Procedure 94 Giving Postmortem Care	Able to Perform	Able to Perform with Assistance	Unable to Perform	Initials and Date
1. Carry out beginning procedure actions. *Comments:*	☐	☐	☐	
2. Assemble equipment. *Comments:*	☐	☐	☐	
3. Apply disposable gloves. *Comments:*	☐	☐	☐	
4. If instructed, remove all appliances, tubing, and used articles. *Comments:*	☐	☐	☐	
5. Work quickly and quietly with respect. *Comments:*	☐	☐	☐	
6. Place the body flat with the head and shoulders elevated on a pillow. *Comments:*	☐	☐	☐	
7. Close the patient's eyes. *Comments:*	☐	☐	☐	
8. Replace dentures in the patient's mouth. *Comments:*	☐	☐	☐	
9. Secure the jaw with light, padded bandaging if necessary. *Comments:*	☐	☐	☐	
10. Straighten the arms and legs and place arms at the sides. *Comments:*	☐	☐	☐	
11. Bathe as necessary. *Comments:*	☐	☐	☐	

continued on the following page

continued from the previous page

Procedure 94	Able to Perform	Able to Perform with Assistance	Unable to Perform	Initials and Date
12. Remove and replace any soiled dressings. *Comments:*	☐	☐	☐	
13. Groom the patient's hair. *Comments:*	☐	☐	☐	
14. Place a disposable pad underneath the buttocks. *Comments:*	☐	☐	☐	
15. If the family is to view the body, put a clean hospital gown on the patient. *Comments:*	☐	☐	☐	
16. Cover the body to the shoulders with a sheet. *Comments:*	☐	☐	☐	
17. Remove and dispose of gloves. *Comments:*	☐	☐	☐	
18. Wash your hands. *Comments:*	☐	☐	☐	
19. Make sure the room is neat and lights are at a subdued level. *Comments:*	☐	☐	☐	
20. Provide chairs and privacy for the family. *Comments:*	☐	☐	☐	
21. After the family leaves, return to the room. Wash your hands and apply disposable gloves. *Comments:*	☐	☐	☐	
22. Collect all belongings and make a list. *Comments:*	☐	☐	☐	
23. Wrap the belongings properly and label, leaving valuables in the hospital safe. *Comments:*	☐	☐	☐	

Procedure 94	Able to Perform	Able to Perform with Assistance	Unable to Perform	Initials and Date
24. Fill out the identification cards or tags in the morgue kit. *Comments:*	☐	☐	☐	
25. Place one card on the right ankle or right great toe. *Comments:*	☐	☐	☐	
26. Attach a card to the bag with the patient's belongings. *Comments:*	☐	☐	☐	
27. Put the shroud on the patient. *Comments:*	☐	☐	☐	
28. Attach an identification card to the outside. *Comments:*	☐	☐	☐	
29. Call an elevator to the floor and keep it empty. *Comments:*	☐	☐	☐	
30. Close patient corridor doors and empty the corridor. *Comments:*	☐	☐	☐	
31. With assistance, place the body on a gurney. *Comments:*	☐	☐	☐	
32. Keep the patient supine. *Comments:*	☐	☐	☐	
33. Cover the body with a sheet. *Comments:*	☐	☐	☐	
34. Remove and dispose of gloves. *Comments:*	☐	☐	☐	
35. Wash your hands. *Comments:*	☐	☐	☐	
36. Take the body to the morgue. *Comments:*	☐	☐	☐	
37. Attach one identification card or tag to the morgue compartment. *Comments:*	☐	☐	☐	

Checklist for Procedure 95   Checking Capillary Refill

Name _____ Date _____

School _____

Instructor _____

Course _____

Procedure 95 Checking Capillary Refill	Able to Perform	Able to Perform with Assistance	Unable to Perform	Initials and Date
1. Carry out beginning procedure actions. *Comments:*	☐	☐	☐	
2. Inspect the nails, noting the color. *Comments:*	☐	☐	☐	
3. Press the nail until the skin underneath turns white. *Comments:*	☐	☐	☐	
4. Release the nail and count the seconds it takes for the skin to return to its normal color. *Comments:*	☐	☐	☐	
5. Carry out procedure completion actions. *Comments:*	☐	☐	☐	

Checklist for Procedure 96   Using a Pulse Oximeter

Name _____ Date _____

School _____

Instructor _____

Course _____

Procedure 96 Using a Pulse Oximeter	Able to Perform	Able to Perform with Assistance	Unable to Perform	Initials and Date
1. Carry out beginning procedure actions. *Comments:*	☐	☐	☐	
2. Assemble equipment. *Comments:*	☐	☐	☐	
3. Select and apply sensor. *Comments:*	☐	☐	☐	
4. Fasten the sensor securely. *Comments:*	☐	☐	☐	
5. Attach the sensor to the patient cable on the pulse oximeter. *Comments:*	☐	☐	☐	
6. Turn the unit on. *Comments:*	☐	☐	☐	
7. Note the percentage of oxygen saturation. *Comments:*	☐	☐	☐	
8. Monitor the patient's pulse rate and respirations. *Comments:*	☐	☐	☐	
9. Inform the nurse and document the readings. *Comments:*	☐	☐	☐	
10. Carry out procedure completion actions. *Comments:*	☐	☐	☐	

Checklist for Procedure 97   Attaching a Humidifier to the Oxygen Flow Meter or Regulator

Name _____ Date _____

School _____

Instructor _____

Course _____

Procedure 97 Attaching a Humidifier to the Oxygen Flow Meter or Regulator	Able to Perform	Able to Perform with Assistance	Unable to Perform	Initials and Date
1. Carry out beginning procedure actions. *Comments:*	☐	☐	☐	
2. Assemble equipment. *Comments:*	☐	☐	☐	
3. Open the humidifier and remove the bottle. *Comments:*	☐	☐	☐	
4. If using a refillable bottle, ensure it has been washed and sterilized. *Comments:*	☐	☐	☐	
5. Unscrew the lid and fill with sterile distilled water. Replace the lid. *Comments:*	☐	☐	☐	
6. Connect the female adapter in the top of the humidifier bottle to the male adapter on the flow meter. *Comments:*	☐	☐	☐	
7. Tighten the nut securely. *Comments:*	☐	☐	☐	
8. Connect the tubing on the cannula or mask to the male adapter on the side of the humidifier bottle. *Comments:*	☐	☐	☐	
9. Turn on the flow of oxygen. *Comments:*	☐	☐	☐	
10. Pinch the connecting tube to ensure that the safety valve pops off. *Comments:*	☐	☐	☐	

continued on the following page

continued from the previous page

Procedure 97	Able to Perform	Able to Perform with Assistance	Unable to Perform	Initials and Date
11. Affix a sticker with the time and date of change and your initials. *Comments:*	☐	☐	☐	
12. Carry out procedure completion actions. *Comments:*	☐	☐	☐	

Checklist for Procedure 98   Collecting a Sputum Specimen

Name _____   Date _____

School _____

Instructor _____

Course _____

Procedure 98 Collecting a Sputum Specimen	Able to Perform	Able to Perform with Assistance	Unable to Perform	Initials and Date
1. Carry out beginning procedure actions. *Comments:*	☐	☐	☐	
2. Assemble equipment. *Comments:*	☐	☐	☐	
3. Wash your hands. *Comments:*	☐	☐	☐	
4. Apply disposable gloves. *Comments:*	☐	☐	☐	
5. Have the patient rinse her mouth with water and spit into an emesis basin. *Comments:*	☐	☐	☐	
6. Instruct the patient to breathe deeply and to cough deeply. *Comments:*	☐	☐	☐	
7. Have the patient spit into a sterile container. *Comments:*	☐	☐	☐	
8. Remove and discard of gloves. *Comments:*	☐	☐	☐	
9. Wash your hands. *Comments:*	☐	☐	☐	
10. Cover the specimen container tightly and attach a completed label. *Comments:*	☐	☐	☐	

continued on the following page

continued from the previous page

Procedure 98	Able to Perform	Able to Perform with Assistance	Unable to Perform	Initials and Date
11. Place the specimen container in a biohazard transport bag and attach a laboratory requisition. *Comments:*	☐	☐	☐	
12. Carry out procedure completion actions. *Comments:*	☐	☐	☐	
13. Transport the specimen to the laboratory according to policy. *Comments:*	☐	☐	☐	

Checklist for Procedure 99 Applying an Arm Sling

Name _____ Date _____

School _____

Instructor _____

Course _____

Procedure 99 Applying an Arm Sling	Able to Perform	Able to Perform with Assistance	Unable to Perform	Initials and Date
1. Carry out beginning procedure actions. *Comments:*	☐	☐	☐	
2. Assemble equipment. *Comments:*	☐	☐	☐	
3. Position affected arm at a 90° angle. *Comments:*	☐	☐	☐	
4. Place one end of the triangle bandage over the unaffected shoulder. *Comments:*	☐	☐	☐	
5. Position the point of the triangle under the affected elbow. *Comments:*	☐	☐	☐	
6. Bring the other end of the triangle over the shoulder on the affected side, covering the arm. *Comments:*	☐	☐	☐	
7. Adjust the bandage so the fingers are elevated. *Comments:*	☐	☐	☐	
8. Tie the ends of the bandage in back. *Comments:*	☐	☐	☐	
9. Position the knot to the side not over the spine. *Comments:*	☐	☐	☐	
10. Pad the skin under the knot. *Comments:*	☐	☐	☐	
11. Fold extra fabric over at the elbow and secure. *Comments:*	☐	☐	☐	

continued on the following page

continued from the previous page

Procedure 99	Able to Perform	Able to Perform with Assistance	Unable to Perform	Initials and Date
12. When applying a commercial sling, support the affected arm and glide the sling up over the hand. *Comments:*	☐	☐	☐	
13. Continue until the elbow is covered and the fingers are exposed. *Comments:*	☐	☐	☐	
14. Wrap the strap around the patient's neck and fasten it to the buckle. *Comments:*	☐	☐	☐	
15. Adjust the strap so the fingers are elevated. *Comments:*	☐	☐	☐	
16. Pad the strap under the neck. *Comments:*	☐	☐	☐	
17. Carry out procedure completion actions. *Comments:*	☐	☐	☐	

Checklist for Procedure 100   Procedure for Continuous Passive Motion

Name _____ Date _____

School _____

Instructor _____

Course _____

Procedure 100 Procedure for Continuous Passive Motion	Able to Perform	Able to Perform with Assistance	Unable to Perform	Initials and Date
1. Carry out beginning procedure actions. *Comments:*	☐	☐	☐	
2. Assemble equipment. *Comments:*	☐	☐	☐	
3. Check the continuous passive motion (CPM) unit for safety and stability. *Comments:*	☐	☐	☐	
4. Have a nurse check the settings. *Comments:*	☐	☐	☐	
5. Stop the CPM unit in full extension. *Comments:*	☐	☐	☐	
6. Raise the side rail on the side where the unit will be. *Comments:*	☐	☐	☐	
7. Position the CPM unit on the bed and secure the attachment. *Comments:*	☐	☐	☐	
8. Fasten the footpad to the footplate with a Velcro fastener. *Comments:*	☐	☐	☐	
9. Attach the tibia/femur sling. *Comments:*	☐	☐	☐	
10. Fasten the Velcro closures under the sling. *Comments:*	☐	☐	☐	
11. Apply the hip pad to the hinge area of the adjustment bar. *Comments:*	☐	☐	☐	

continued on the following page

continued from the previous page

Procedure 100	Able to Perform	Able to Perform with Assistance	Unable to Perform	Initials and Date
12. Position the femur sling straps over the hinges. Fasten underneath with Velcro. *Comments:*	☐	☐	☐	
13. Fit the CPM unit to the patient's leg length. *Comments:*	☐	☐	☐	
14. Align the knee joint with the knee hinge. *Comments:*	☐	☐	☐	
15. Position the knee approximately 1 inch below the knee joint line. *Comments:*	☐	☐	☐	
16. Center the leg on the unit. *Comments:*	☐	☐	☐	
17. Adjust the footpad. *Comments:*	☐	☐	☐	
18. Secure the Velcro straps across the thigh and top of foot. *Comments:*	☐	☐	☐	
19. Give the patient the control and instruct the patient in starting the unit. *Comments:*	☐	☐	☐	
20. Stay with the patient for two full cycles. *Comments:*	☐	☐	☐	
21. Return to check on the patient frequently. *Comments:*	☐	☐	☐	
22. Document any information if necessary. *Comments:*	☐	☐	☐	
23. Carry out procedure completion actions. *Comments:*	☐	☐	☐	

Checklist for Procedure 101   Performing Range-of-Motion Exercises (Passive)

Name _____ Date _____

School _____

Instructor _____

Course _____

Procedure 101 **Performing Range-of-Motion Exercises (Passive)**	Able to Perform	Able to Perform with Assistance	Unable to Perform	Initials and Date
1. Carry out beginning procedure actions. *Comments:*	☐	☐	☐	
2. Assemble equipment. *Comments:*	☐	☐	☐	
3. Position the patient on his back. *Comments:*	☐	☐	☐	
4. Adjust the bath blanket to keep the patient covered. *Comments:*	☐	☐	☐	
5. Support the elbow and wrist. *Comments:*	☐	☐	☐	
6. To exercise the shoulder joint, bring the entire arm out at a right angle to the body. *Comments:*	☐	☐	☐	
7. Return the arm to a position parallel to the body. *Comments:*	☐	☐	☐	
8. Roll the entire arm toward the body. *Comments:*	☐	☐	☐	
9. Roll the entire arm away from the body. *Comments:*	☐	☐	☐	
10. With the shoulder in abduction, flex the elbow and raise the entire arm over the head. *Comments:*	☐	☐	☐	

continued on the following page

continued from the previous page

Procedure 101	Able to Perform	Able to Perform with Assistance	Unable to Perform	Initials and Date
11. With arm parallel to the body, flex and extend the elbow. *Comments:*	☐	☐	☐	
12. Flex and extend the wrist. *Comments:*	☐	☐	☐	
13. Flex and extend each finger joint. *Comments:*	☐	☐	☐	
14. Move each finger away from the middle finger and toward the middle finger. *Comments:*	☐	☐	☐	
15. Abduct the thumb by moving it toward the extended fingers. *Comments:*	☐	☐	☐	
16. Touch the thumb to the base of the little finger, then to each fingertip. *Comments:*	☐	☐	☐	
17. Turn the hand palm down, then palm up. *Comments:*	☐	☐	☐	
18. Grasp the patient's wrist with one hand and the patient's hand with the other. *Comments:*	☐	☐	☐	
19. Bring the wrist toward the body and then away from the body. *Comments:*	☐	☐	☐	
20. Point the hand in supination toward the thumb side, then toward the little-finger side. *Comments:*	☐	☐	☐	
21. Cover the patient's upper extremities and body. *Comments:*	☐	☐	☐	

Procedure 101	Able to Perform	Able to Perform with Assistance	Unable to Perform	Initials and Date
22. Expose only the leg being exercised. *Comments:*	☐	☐	☐	
23. Face the foot of the bed. *Comments:*	☐	☐	☐	
24. Support the knee and ankle and then move the entire leg away from the body center and toward the body. *Comments:*	☐	☐	☐	
25. Turn to face the bed. *Comments:*	☐	☐	☐	
26. Support the knee in bent position. Raise the knee toward the pelvis. *Comments:*	☐	☐	☐	
27. Straighten the knee as you lower the leg to the bed. *Comments:*	☐	☐	☐	
28. Support the leg at the knee and ankle; then roll the leg in a circular fashion away from the body. *Comments:*	☐	☐	☐	
29. Continue to support the leg and roll the leg in the same fashion toward the body. *Comments:*	☐	☐	☐	
30. Grasp the patient's toes and support the ankle. *Comments:*	☐	☐	☐	
31. Bring the toes toward the knee. *Comments:*	☐	☐	☐	
32. Point the toes toward the foot of the bed. *Comments:*	☐	☐	☐	
33. Gently turn the patient's foot inward and outward. *Comments:*	☐	☐	☐	

continued on the following page

continued from the previous page

Procedure 101	Able to Perform	Able to Perform with Assistance	Unable to Perform	Initials and Date
34. Place your fingers over the patient's toes. *Comments:*	☐	☐	☐	
35. Bend the toes and straighten them. *Comments:*	☐	☐	☐	
36. Move each toe away from the second toe and then toward the second toe. *Comments:*	☐	☐	☐	
37. Cover the leg with the bath blanket. *Comments:*	☐	☐	☐	
38. Raise the side rail and move to the opposite side of the bed. *Comments:*	☐	☐	☐	
39. Move the patient close to you and repeat steps 5–36. *Comments:*	☐	☐	☐	
40. Carry out procedure completion actions. *Comments:*	☐	☐	☐	

Checklist for Procedure 102   Obtaining a Fingerstick Blood Sugar

Name _____   Date _____

School _____

Instructor _____

Course _____

Procedure 102 Obtaining a Fingerstick Blood Sugar	Able to Perform	Able to Perform with Assistance	Unable to Perform	Initials and Date
1. Carry out beginning procedure actions. *Comments:*	☐	☐	☐	
2. Assemble equipment. *Comments:*	☐	☐	☐	
3. Wipe the patient's finger with an alcohol sponge and allow it to dry. *Comments:*	☐	☐	☐	
4. Pierce the sides of the middle or ring finger with a lancet. *Comments:*	☐	☐	☐	
5. Discard the lancet into a sharps container. *Comments:*	☐	☐	☐	
6. Gently squeeze the sides of the finger. *Comments:*	☐	☐	☐	
7. Hold the puncture site directly over the reagent. *Comments:*	☐	☐	☐	
8. Place a hanging drop of blood onto the reagent pad. *Comments:*	☐	☐	☐	
9. If using capillary tube strips, peel the package back to open. *Comments:*	☐	☐	☐	
10. Hold the package firmly, with your thumb and forefinger over the test end of the strip. *Comments:*	☐	☐	☐	

continued on the following page

continued from the previous page

Procedure 102	Able to Perform	Able to Perform with Assistance	Unable to Perform	Initials and Date
11. Insert the strip into the meter. *Comments:*	☐	☐	☐	
12. Remove and discard the package. *Comments:*	☐	☐	☐	
13. Hold the strip next to the puncture site to draw blood into the straw. *Comments:*	☐	☐	☐	
14. Insert the strip into the meter. *Comments:*	☐	☐	☐	
15. Wipe the patient's finger with an alcohol sponge and allow it to dry. *Comments:*	☐	☐	☐	
16. Apply pressure until bleeding stops and apply a bandage strip. *Comments:*	☐	☐	☐	
17. Read the meter after the designated period of time. *Comments:*	☐	☐	☐	
18. Carry out procedure completion actions. *Comments:*	☐	☐	☐	

Checklist for Procedure 103   Testing Urine for Acetone: Ketostix® Strip Test

Name _____ Date _____

School _____

Instructor _____

Course _____

Procedure 103 Testing Urine for Acetone: Ketostix® Strip Test	Able to Perform	Able to Perform with Assistance	Unable to Perform	Initials and Date
1. Carry out beginning procedure actions. Comments:	☐	☐	☐	
2. Assemble equipment. Comments:	☐	☐	☐	
3. Apply disposable gloves. Comments:	☐	☐	☐	
4. Remove test strip from the bottle and recap. Comments:	☐	☐	☐	
5. Dip one end of the test strip into the fresh urine sample. Comments:	☐	☐	☐	
6. Remove strip and hold horizontally. Comments:	☐	☐	☐	
7. After 15 seconds, compare the strip with the color chart on the bottle label. Comments:	☐	☐	☐	
8. Match as closely as possible to one of the colors on the chart. Comments:	☐	☐	☐	
9. Dispose of the strip and urine specimen unless there are orders to save them. Comments:	☐	☐	☐	
10. Remove and dispose of gloves. Comments:	☐	☐	☐	
11. Carry out procedure completion actions. Comments:	☐	☐	☐	

Checklist for Procedure 104   Caring for the Eye Socket and Artificial Eye

Name _____ Date _____

School _____

Instructor _____

Course _____

Procedure 104 **Caring for the Eye Socket and Artificial Eye**	Able to Perform	Able to Perform with Assistance	Unable to Perform	Initials and Date
1. Carry out beginning procedure actions. *Comments:*	☐	☐	☐	
2. Assemble equipment. *Comments:*	☐	☐	☐	
3. Place the patient in supine position if tolerated. *Comments:*	☐	☐	☐	
4. Place a towel across the patient's chest. *Comments:*	☐	☐	☐	
5. Apply disposable gloves. *Comments:*	☐	☐	☐	
6. Moisten cotton balls in lukewarm water. *Comments:*	☐	☐	☐	
7. Ask the patient to close his eyes. *Comments:*	☐	☐	☐	
8. Wipe the upper lid of the affected eye from the inner corner of the eye to the outer edge. *Comments:*	☐	☐	☐	
9. Repeat with a clean cotton ball until area is clean. *Comments:*	☐	☐	☐	
10. Dispose of used cotton balls. *Comments:*	☐	☐	☐	

continued on the following page

continued from the previous page

Procedure 104	Able to Perform	Able to Perform with Assistance	Unable to Perform	Initials and Date
11. Place a 4 × 4 pad in the bottom of an eyecup or denture cup. *Comments:*	☐	☐	☐	
12. Gently pull down the lower eyelid with your thumb. *Comments:*	☐	☐	☐	
13. Open the upper lid with your index finger. *Comments:*	☐	☐	☐	
14. Grasp the artificial eye as it comes out of the eye socket. *Comments:*	☐	☐	☐	
15. Place it on the gauze in the cup. *Comments:*	☐	☐	☐	
16. If a suction cup is used, gently hold the eye open with the fingers of one hand. *Comments:*	☐	☐	☐	
17. Depress the suction cup between your thumb and index finger. *Comments:*	☐	☐	☐	
18. Place the suction cup in the center of the artificial eye. *Comments:*	☐	☐	☐	
19. Release the pressure. *Comments:*	☐	☐	☐	
20. Gently pull the eye from the socket. *Comments:*	☐	☐	☐	
21. Clean the empty eye socket with clean, moist cotton balls. *Comments:*	☐	☐	☐	
22. Dry gently with clean, dry cotton balls. *Comments:*	☐	☐	☐	

Procedure 104	Able to Perform	Able to Perform with Assistance	Unable to Perform	Initials and Date
23. Carry the cup with the artificial eye to the sink. *Comments:*	☐	☐	☐	
24. Fill the sink one-third full with lukewarm water. *Comments:*	☐	☐	☐	
25. Wash the eye under lukewarm running water. *Comments:*	☐	☐	☐	
26. Rinse the eye and place it on a 4 × 4 gauze pad. *Comments:*	☐	☐	☐	
27. Store the eye according to care plan. *Comments:*	☐	☐	☐	
28. Discard the water or solution in the eyecup and rinse the cup. *Comments:*	☐	☐	☐	
29. Remove and dispose of gloves. *Comments:*	☐	☐	☐	
30. Wash your hands. *Comments:*	☐	☐	☐	
31. Carry the artificial eye to the patient's bedside. *Comments:*	☐	☐	☐	
32. To insert the artificial eye, carry out beginning procedure actions. *Comments:*	☐	☐	☐	
33. Apply disposable gloves. *Comments:*	☐	☐	☐	
34. Clean and rinse the artificial eye. *Comments:*	☐	☐	☐	
35. Position the notched edge of the eye toward the patient's nose. *Comments:*	☐	☐	☐	

continued on the following page

continued from the previous page

Procedure 104	Able to Perform	Able to Perform with Assistance	Unable to Perform	Initials and Date
36. Gently open the upper lid. *Comments:*	☐	☐	☐	
37. Bring the prosthesis up past the lower lid and under the upper lid. *Comments:*	☐	☐	☐	
38. Set it flush once it is past the lower lid and touching the upper tissues. *Comments:*	☐	☐	☐	
39. Use your index finger to slip it up under the upper lid. *Comments:*	☐	☐	☐	
40. Release the upper lid. *Comments:*	☐	☐	☐	
41. Draw the edge of the lower lid forward, covering the lower edge of the eye and press down lightly. *Comments:*	☐	☐	☐	
42. Carry out procedure completion actions. *Comments:*	☐	☐	☐	

Checklist for Procedure 105   Warm Eye Compresses

Name _____   Date _____

School _____

Instructor _____

Course _____

Procedure 105 Warm Eye Compresses	Able to Perform	Able to Perform with Assistance	Unable to Perform	Initials and Date
1. Carry out beginning procedure actions. *Comments:*	☐	☐	☐	
2. Assemble equipment. *Comments:*	☐	☐	☐	
3. Assist the patient to a Fowler's or high Fowler's position if possible. *Comments:*	☐	☐	☐	
4. Cover the neck and shoulders with a bath towel. *Comments:*	☐	☐	☐	
5. Heat the bottle of sterile saline. *Comments:*	☐	☐	☐	
6. Check for a temperature of approximately 105°F. *Comments:*	☐	☐	☐	
7. Pour the heated saline into a small, sterile bowl. *Comments:*	☐	☐	☐	
8. Wash your hands. *Comments:*	☐	☐	☐	
9. Apply disposable gloves. *Comments:*	☐	☐	☐	
10. Place gauze pads in the bowl of saline. *Comments:*	☐	☐	☐	
11. Remove one pad and squeeze out excess saline. *Comments:*	☐	☐	☐	

continued on the following page

continued from the previous page

Procedure 105	Able to Perform	Able to Perform with Assistance	Unable to Perform	Initials and Date
12. Instruct the patient to close her eyes. *Comments:*	☐	☐	☐	
13. Apply one compress to affected eye. *Comments:*	☐	☐	☐	
14. Remove the second pad and squeeze out excess saline. *Comments:*	☐	☐	☐	
15. Apply the second compress on top of the first. *Comments:*	☐	☐	☐	
16. Repeat with the other eye, as directed. *Comments:*	☐	☐	☐	
17. Change the compresses every few minutes, checking the skin underneath. *Comments:*	☐	☐	☐	
18. Treat for 15 to 20 minutes; remove and discard the compresses. *Comments:*	☐	☐	☐	
19. Dry the eye with clean gauze pads. *Comments:*	☐	☐	☐	
20. Carry out procedure completion actions. *Comments:*	☐	☐	☐	

Checklist for Procedure 106   Cool Eye Compresses

Name _____ Date _____

School _____

Instructor _____

Course _____

Procedure 106 Cool Eye Compresses	Able to Perform	Able to Perform with Assistance	Unable to Perform	Initials and Date
1. Carry out beginning procedure actions. *Comments:*	☐	☐	☐	
2. Assemble equipment. *Comments:*	☐	☐	☐	
3. Place the patient in supine position. *Comments:*	☐	☐	☐	
4. Turn the patient's head slightly, affected eye up. *Comments:*	☐	☐	☐	
5. Cover the neck and shoulders with a bath towel. *Comments:*	☐	☐	☐	
6. Place ice chips in a small, sterile basin. *Comments:*	☐	☐	☐	
7. Pour saline solution into the basin. *Comments:*	☐	☐	☐	
8. Wash your hands. *Comments:*	☐	☐	☐	
9. Apply disposable gloves. *Comments:*	☐	☐	☐	
10. Place gauze pads in the bowl of saline. *Comments:*	☐	☐	☐	
11. Remove one pad and squeeze out excess saline. *Comments:*	☐	☐	☐	

continued on the following page

continued from the previous page

Procedure 106	Able to Perform	Able to Perform with Assistance	Unable to Perform	Initials and Date
12. Instruct the patient to close his eyes. *Comments:*	☐	☐	☐	
13. Apply one compress to affected eye. *Comments:*	☐	☐	☐	
14. Remove the second pad and squeeze out excess saline. *Comments:*	☐	☐	☐	
15. Apply the second compress on top of the first. *Comments:*	☐	☐	☐	
16. Repeat with the other eye, as directed. *Comments:*	☐	☐	☐	
17. If the compress is too cold, remove it immediately. *Comments:*	☐	☐	☐	
18. If an ice pack is to be used, make it by placing ice chips in a small sandwich bag or disposable glove and cover the compress. *Comments:*	☐	☐	☐	
19. Change the compresses every few minutes, checking the skin underneath. *Comments:*	☐	☐	☐	
20. Treat for 15 to 20 minutes; remove and discard the compresses. *Comments:*	☐	☐	☐	
21. Dry the eye with clean gauze pads. *Comments:*	☐	☐	☐	
22. Carry out procedure completion actions. *Comments:*	☐	☐	☐	

Checklist for Procedure 107   Applying a Behind-the-Ear Hearing Aid

Name _____ Date _____

School _____

Instructor _____

Course _____

Procedure 107 Applying a Behind-the-Ear Hearing Aid	Able to Perform	Able to Perform with Assistance	Unable to Perform	Initials and Date
1. Carry out beginning procedure actions. *Comments:*	☐	☐	☐	
2. Assemble equipment. *Comments:*	☐	☐	☐	
3. Check that the hearing aid is in working order. *Comments:*	☐	☐	☐	
4. Check that the appliance is off and the volume is turned to its lowest level. *Comments:*	☐	☐	☐	
5. Check the patient's ear for wax buildup. *Comments:*	☐	☐	☐	
6. Carefully hand the hearing aid to the patient, supporting it as he inserts the ear mold into the ear canal. *Comments:*	☐	☐	☐	
7. If assistance is needed, place the hearing aid over the patient's ear. *Comments:*	☐	☐	☐	
8. Allow the ear mold to hang free. *Comments:*	☐	☐	☐	
9. Adjust the hearing aid behind the patient's ear. *Comments:*	☐	☐	☐	
10. Grasp the ear mold and gently insert the tapered end into the ear canal. *Comments:*	☐	☐	☐	

continued on the following page

continued from the previous page

Procedure 107	Able to Perform	Able to Perform with Assistance	Unable to Perform	Initials and Date
11. Gently twist the ear mold into the curve of the ear. *Comments:*	☐	☐	☐	
12. Turn on the control switch and adjust the volume. *Comments:*	☐	☐	☐	
13. Carry out procedure completion actions. *Comments:*	☐	☐	☐	

Checklist for Procedure 108   Removing a Behind-the-Ear Hearing Aid

Name _____ Date _____

School _____

Instructor _____

Course _____

Procedure 108 Removing a Behind-the-Ear Hearing Aid	Able to Perform	Able to Perform with Assistance	Unable to Perform	Initials and Date
1. Carry out beginning procedure actions. *Comments:*	☐	☐	☐	
2. Explain the procedure to the patient. *Comments:*	☐	☐	☐	
3. Turn off the hearing aid. *Comments:*	☐	☐	☐	
4. Loosen the outer portion of the ear mold by gently pulling on the upper part of the ear. *Comments:*	☐	☐	☐	
5. Lift the ear mold upward and outward. *Comments:*	☐	☐	☐	
6. Double check the hearing aid to ensure the switch is in the off position. *Comments:*	☐	☐	☐	
7. Carry out procedure completion actions. *Comments:*	☐	☐	☐	

Checklist for Procedure 109 Applying and Removing an In-the-Ear Hearing Aid

Name _____ Date _____

School _____

Instructor _____

Course _____

Procedure 109 Applying and Removing an In-the-Ear Hearing Aid	Able to Perform	Able to Perform with Assistance	Unable to Perform	Initials and Date
1. Carry out beginning procedure actions. *Comments:*	☐	☐	☐	
2. Assemble equipment. *Comments:*	☐	☐	☐	
3. Turn the hearing aid off and the volume down. *Comments:*	☐	☐	☐	
4. Grasp the ear mold and gently insert the tapered end into the ear canal. *Comments:*	☐	☐	☐	
5. Gently twist the ear mold into the curve of the ear while gently pulling on the ear lobe with your other hand. *Comments:*	☐	☐	☐	
6. Turn on the control switch. *Comments:*	☐	☐	☐	
7. Talk to the patient as you increase the volume; stop when the patient can hear you. *Comments:*	☐	☐	☐	
8. To remove the hearing aid, wash your hands and explain what you are going to do. *Comments:*	☐	☐	☐	
9. Turn off the hearing aid. *Comments:*	☐	☐	☐	
10. Gently pull on the upper part of the ear to loosen the outer portion of the ear mold. *Comments:*	☐	☐	☐	

continued on the following page

continued from the previous page

Procedure 109	Able to Perform	Able to Perform with Assistance	Unable to Perform	Initials and Date
11. Lift the ear mold upward and outward. *Comments:*	☐	☐	☐	
12. Store the aid in a safe area either without the batteries or with the battery compartment open. *Comments:*	☐	☐	☐	
13. Carry out procedure completion actions. *Comments:*	☐	☐	☐	

Checklist for Procedure 110   Collecting a Stool Specimen

Name _____ Date _____

School _____

Instructor _____

Course _____

Procedure 110 **Collecting a Stool Specimen**	Able to Perform	Able to Perform with Assistance	Unable to Perform	Initials and Date
1. Carry out beginning procedure actions. *Comments:*	☐	☐	☐	
2. Assemble equipment. *Comments:*	☐	☐	☐	
3. Wash your hands. *Comments:*	☐	☐	☐	
4. Apply disposable gloves. *Comments:*	☐	☐	☐	
5. If the patient is incontinent of feces, collect the specimen from bed linens or diaper. *Comments:*	☐	☐	☐	
6. Assist the patient to use a bedpan or bedside commode. *Comments:*	☐	☐	☐	
7. Help the patient to wash hands and perform perineal care if necessary. *Comments:*	☐	☐	☐	
8. Take the collection container to the bathroom and use tongue blades to remove a specimen. *Comments:*	☐	☐	☐	
9. Place the specimen in a specimen container. *Comments:*	☐	☐	☐	
10. Empty the collection container into the toilet and clean or dispose of it. *Comments:*	☐	☐	☐	

continued on the following page

continued from the previous page

Procedure 110	Able to Perform	Able to Perform with Assistance	Unable to Perform	Initials and Date
11. Remove and dispose of gloves. *Comments:*	☐	☐	☐	
12. Place cover tightly on the specimen container and attach completed label. *Comments:*	☐	☐	☐	
13. Place the container in a biohazard transport bag. *Comments:*	☐	☐	☐	
14. Promptly take or send the specimen to the laboratory. *Comments:*	☐	☐	☐	
15. Carry out procedure completion actions. *Comments:*	☐	☐	☐	

Checklist for Procedure 111   Giving a Soap-Solution Enema

Name _____ Date _____

School _____

Instructor _____

Course _____

Procedure 111 Giving a Soap-Solution Enema	Able to Perform	Able to Perform with Assistance	Unable to Perform	Initials and Date
1. Carry out beginning procedure actions. *Comments:*	☐	☐	☐	
2. Assemble equipment. *Comments:*	☐	☐	☐	
3. Connect the tubing to the solution container. *Comments:*	☐	☐	☐	
4. Adjust the clamp on the tubing and snap it shut. *Comments:*	☐	☐	☐	
5. Fill the container with warm water to the 1,000-mL line. *Comments:*	☐	☐	☐	
6. Put the liquid soap in the water. *Comments:*	☐	☐	☐	
7. Gently mix the solution. *Comments:*	☐	☐	☐	
8. Run a small amount of solution through the tube. *Comments:*	☐	☐	☐	
9. Clamp the tubing. *Comments:*	☐	☐	☐	
10. Place a chair at the foot of the bed and cover with a bed protector. *Comments:*	☐	☐	☐	
11. Place the bedpan on the chair. *Comments:*	☐	☐	☐	

continued on the following page

continued from the previous page

Procedure 111	Able to Perform	Able to Perform with Assistance	Unable to Perform	Initials and Date
12. Elevate the bed to a comfortable working height. *Comments:*	☐	☐	☐	
13. Raise the opposite side rail and secure. *Comments:*	☐	☐	☐	
14. Cover the patient with a bath blanket and fanfold linen to the foot of the bed. *Comments:*	☐	☐	☐	
15. Wash your hands and apply disposable gloves. *Comments:*	☐	☐	☐	
16. Place a bed protector under the patient's buttocks. *Comments:*	☐	☐	☐	
17. Assist the patient to turn to his left side and flex the knees. *Comments:*	☐	☐	☐	
18. Place the container of solution on the chair so tubing will reach the patient. *Comments:*	☐	☐	☐	
19. Expose the anal area. *Comments:*	☐	☐	☐	
20. Lubricate the tip of the tube. *Comments:*	☐	☐	☐	
21. Instruct the patient to breathe deeply and bear down as the tube is inserted. *Comments:*	☐	☐	☐	
22. Insert the tube 2 to 4 inches into the anus. Never force the tube. *Comments:*	☐	☐	☐	
23. Open the clamp and raise the container 12 inches above the level of the anus. *Comments:*	☐	☐	☐	
24. Ask the patient to take deep breaths to relax the abdomen. *Comments:*	☐	☐	☐	

Procedure 111	Able to Perform	Able to Perform with Assistance	Unable to Perform	Initials and Date
25. If patient has cramping, stop the procedure until cramping stops. *Comments:*	☐	☐	☐	
26. Clamp the tubing before the container is completely empty. *Comments:*	☐	☐	☐	
27. Have the patient hold his breath while you raise the upper buttock and gently withdraw the tube. *Comments:*	☐	☐	☐	
28. Wrap the tubing in a paper towel and put in a disposable container. *Comments:*	☐	☐	☐	
29. Place patient on a bedpan or assist him to the bathroom. *Comments:*	☐	☐	☐	
30. If patient uses the bedpan, raise the head of the bed to a comfortable height and raise the side rail. *Comments:*	☐	☐	☐	
31. Place toilet tissue and the call signal within the patient's reach. *Comments:*	☐	☐	☐	
32. Remove and dispose of gloves. *Comments:*	☐	☐	☐	
33. Wash your hands. *Comments:*	☐	☐	☐	
34. When the patient is finished, return to the bedside and apply fresh gloves. *Comments:*	☐	☐	☐	
35. Lower the side rail. *Comments:*	☐	☐	☐	
36. Remove the bedpan, place on the covered chair, and cover. *Comments:*	☐	☐	☐	
37. Cleanse the anal area. *Comments:*	☐	☐	☐	

continued on the following page

continued from the previous page

Procedure 111	Able to Perform	Able to Perform with Assistance	Unable to Perform	Initials and Date
38. Remove the bed protector and discard. *Comments:*	☐	☐	☐	
39. Remove and dispose of gloves. *Comments:*	☐	☐	☐	
40. Wash your hands. *Comments:*	☐	☐	☐	
41. If the patient uses the bathroom, stay nearby and caution him not to flush the toilet. *Comments:*	☐	☐	☐	
42. Give the patient soap, water, and towel to wash and dry his hands. *Comments:*	☐	☐	☐	
43. Replace the top bedding and remove the bath blanket. *Comments:*	☐	☐	☐	
44. Apply disposable gloves. *Comments:*	☐	☐	☐	
45. Take the bedpan to the bathroom and dispose of the contents. *Comments:*	☐	☐	☐	
46. Remove and dispose of gloves. *Comments:*	☐	☐	☐	
47. Wash your hands. *Comments:*	☐	☐	☐	
48. Air the room and leave the room in order. *Comments:*	☐	☐	☐	
49. Unscreen the unit. *Comments:*	☐	☐	☐	
50. Clean and replace all equipment according to policy. *Comments:*	☐	☐	☐	
51. Carry out procedure completion actions. *Comments:*	☐	☐	☐	

Checklist for Procedure 112   Giving a Commercially Prepared Enema

Name _____ Date _____

School _____

Instructor _____

Course _____

Procedure 112 Giving a Commercially Prepared Enema	Able to Perform	Able to Perform with Assistance	Unable to Perform	Initials and Date
1. Carry out beginning procedure actions. *Comments:*	☐	☐	☐	
2. Assemble equipment. *Comments:*	☐	☐	☐	
3. Open the package and remove the plastic container of enema solution. *Comments:*	☐	☐	☐	
4. Place the solution container in warm water. *Comments:*	☐	☐	☐	
5. Lower the head of the bed to a horizontal position. *Comments:*	☐	☐	☐	
6. Elevate the bed to a comfortable working height. *Comments:*	☐	☐	☐	
7. Raise the opposite side rail. *Comments:*	☐	☐	☐	
8. Apply disposable gloves. *Comments:*	☐	☐	☐	
9. Place a bedpan and cover on the chair close at hand. *Comments:*	☐	☐	☐	
10. Assist the patient to turn to the left side and flex the right leg. *Comments:*	☐	☐	☐	
11. Place a bed protector under the patient. *Comments:*	☐	☐	☐	

continued on the following page

continued from the previous page

Procedure 112	Able to Perform	Able to Perform with Assistance	Unable to Perform	Initials and Date
12. Expose the patient's buttocks. *Comments:*	☐	☐	☐	
13. Remove the cover from the enema tip. *Comments:*	☐	☐	☐	
14. Gently squeeze to check the tip for damage. *Comments:*	☐	☐	☐	
15. Separate the buttocks, exposing the anus. *Comments:*	☐	☐	☐	
16. Instruct the patient to breathe deeply and bear down as the enema tip is inserted. *Comments:*	☐	☐	☐	
17. Insert the lubricated tip 2 inches into the rectum. *Comments:*	☐	☐	☐	
18. Gently squeeze and roll the container until desired quantity of solution is administered. *Comments:*	☐	☐	☐	
19. Remove the tip from the patient and place the container in the box. *Comments:*	☐	☐	☐	
20. Encourage the patient to hold the solution as long as possible. *Comments:*	☐	☐	☐	
21. Remove and dispose of gloves. *Comments:*	☐	☐	☐	
22. Wash your hands. *Comments:*	☐	☐	☐	
23. Discard the used enema as biohazard waste. *Comments:*	☐	☐	☐	

Procedure 112	Able to Perform	Able to Perform with Assistance	Unable to Perform	Initials and Date
24. Give the patient the call signal and leave. *Comments:*	☐	☐	☐	
25. When the patient signals, return to the room and lower the bed. *Comments:*	☐	☐	☐	
26. Assist the patient to the bathroom or position the patient on a bedpan. *Comments:*	☐	☐	☐	
27. Raise the head of the bed if patient is using a bedpan. *Comments:*	☐	☐	☐	
28. Place toilet tissue and the call signal within the patient's reach. *Comments:*	☐	☐	☐	
29. Raise the side rail. *Comments:*	☐	☐	☐	
30. Return when signaled and wash your hands. *Comments:*	☐	☐	☐	
31. Lower the side rail. *Comments:*	☐	☐	☐	
32. Apply disposable gloves. *Comments:*	☐	☐	☐	
33. Remove the bedpan and place it on the covered chair. *Comments:*	☐	☐	☐	
34. Observe the contents and cover the bedpan. *Comments:*	☐	☐	☐	
35. Clean the anal area if necessary. *Comments:*	☐	☐	☐	
36. Take the bedpan and equipment to the bathroom. *Comments:*	☐	☐	☐	

continued on the following page

continued from the previous page

Procedure 112	Able to Perform	Able to Perform with Assistance	Unable to Perform	Initials and Date
37. Dispose of contents according to policy. *Comments:*	☐	☐	☐	
38. Remove and dispose of gloves. *Comments:*	☐	☐	☐	
39. If the patient uses the bathroom, stay nearby and caution him not to flush the toilet. *Comments:*	☐	☐	☐	
40. Apply disposable gloves. *Comments:*	☐	☐	☐	
41. Clean the anal area if necessary. *Comments:*	☐	☐	☐	
42. Observe the contents of the toilet. *Comments:*	☐	☐	☐	
43. Flush the toilet or cover it. *Comments:*	☐	☐	☐	
44. Remove and dispose of gloves. *Comments:*	☐	☐	☐	
45. Assist the patient into bed. *Comments:*	☐	☐	☐	
46. Give the patient soap, water, and towel to wash and dry his hands. *Comments:*	☐	☐	☐	
47. Leave the side rails down unless needed for safety and leave the bed in the low position. *Comments:*	☐	☐	☐	
48. Carry out procedure completion actions. *Comments:*	☐	☐	☐	

Checklist for Procedure 113   Inserting a Rectal Suppository

Name _____ Date _____

School _____

Instructor _____

Course _____

Procedure 113 Inserting a Rectal Suppository	Able to Perform	Able to Perform with Assistance	Unable to Perform	Initials and Date
1. Carry out beginning procedure actions. *Comments:*	☐	☐	☐	
2. Assemble equipment. *Comments:*	☐	☐	☐	
3. Wash your hands. *Comments:*	☐	☐	☐	
4. Apply disposable gloves. *Comments:*	☐	☐	☐	
5. Assist the patient to turn on left side and flex the right leg. *Comments:*	☐	☐	☐	
6. Place a bed protector under the patient's hips. *Comments:*	☐	☐	☐	
7. Expose the patient's buttocks. *Comments:*	☐	☐	☐	
8. Unwrap the suppository. *Comments:*	☐	☐	☐	
9. Separate the patient's buttocks to expose the anus. *Comments:*	☐	☐	☐	
10. Apply a small amount of lubricant to the anus and the suppository. *Comments:*	☐	☐	☐	
11. Insert the suppository approximately 2 inches. *Comments:*	☐	☐	☐	

continued on the following page

continued from the previous page

Procedure 113	Able to Perform	Able to Perform with Assistance	Unable to Perform	Initials and Date
12. Encourage the patient to take deep breaths and relax. *Comments:*	☐	☐	☐	
13. Remove and dispose of gloves. *Comments:*	☐	☐	☐	
14. Wash your hands. *Comments:*	☐	☐	☐	
15. Help the patient into a comfortable position and leave the call signal within the patient's reach. *Comments:*	☐	☐	☐	
16. Check the patient every 5 minutes. *Comments:*	☐	☐	☐	
17. When the patient feels the need to defecate, wash your hands and apply disposable gloves. *Comments:*	☐	☐	☐	
18. Assist the patient to the bathroom or commode, or position the patient on a bedpan and provide privacy. *Comments:*	☐	☐	☐	
19. When the patient is finished, assist with hygiene if necessary. *Comments:*	☐	☐	☐	
20. Observe the results and report any unusual characteristics to the nurse. *Comments:*	☐	☐	☐	
21. Dispose of stool and clean equipment. *Comments:*	☐	☐	☐	
22. Remove and dispose of gloves. *Comments:*	☐	☐	☐	
23. Wash your hands. *Comments:*	☐	☐	☐	
24. Carry out procedure completion actions. *Comments:*	☐	☐	☐	

Checklist for Procedure 114   Inserting a Rectal Tube and Flatus Bag

Name _____ Date _____

School _____

Instructor _____

Course _____

Procedure 114 **Inserting a Rectal Tube and Flatus Bag**	Able to Perform	Able to Perform with Assistance	Unable to Perform	Initials and Date
1. Carry out beginning procedure actions. *Comments:*	☐	☐	☐	
2. Assemble equipment. *Comments:*	☐	☐	☐	
3. Identify the patient and screen the unit. *Comments:*	☐	☐	☐	
4. Explain what you plan to do. *Comments:*	☐	☐	☐	
5. Lower the head of the bed to the horizontal position. *Comments:*	☐	☐	☐	
6. Wash your hands. *Comments:*	☐	☐	☐	
7. Apply disposable gloves. *Comments:*	☐	☐	☐	
8. Assist the patient to turn to the left side and flex the right leg. *Comments:*	☐	☐	☐	
9. Place a bed protector under the hips. *Comments:*	☐	☐	☐	
10. Expose the patient's buttocks. *Comments:*	☐	☐	☐	
11. Lubricate the tip of the rectal tube. *Comments:*	☐	☐	☐	
12. Separate the buttocks to expose the anus. *Comments:*	☐	☐	☐	

continued on the following page

continued from the previous page

Procedure 114	Able to Perform	Able to Perform with Assistance	Unable to Perform	Initials and Date
13. Instruct the patient to breathe deeply and bear down gently. *Comments:*	☐	☐	☐	
14. Insert the lubricated rectal tube 2 to 4 inches. *Comments:*	☐	☐	☐	
15. Secure the rectal tube in place. *Comments:*	☐	☐	☐	
16. Remove and dispose of gloves. *Comments:*	☐	☐	☐	
17. Help the patient into a comfortable position and leave the call signal within the patient's reach. *Comments:*	☐	☐	☐	
18. Return to the unit in 20 minutes. *Comments:*	☐	☐	☐	
19. Wash your hands. *Comments:*	☐	☐	☐	
20. Apply disposable gloves. *Comments:*	☐	☐	☐	
21. Gently remove the rectal tube. *Comments:*	☐	☐	☐	
22. Place the rectal tube on a paper towel. *Comments:*	☐	☐	☐	
23. Clean the area around the anus. *Comments:*	☐	☐	☐	
24. Dispose of the wrapped rectal tube and bag. *Comments:*	☐	☐	☐	
25. Remove and dispose of gloves. *Comments:*	☐	☐	☐	
26. Wash your hands. *Comments:*	☐	☐	☐	
27. Carry out procedure completion actions. *Comments:*	☐	☐	☐	

Checklist for Procedure 115   Collecting a Routine Urine Specimen

Name _____   Date _____

School _____

Instructor _____

Course _____

Procedure 115 Collecting a Routine Urine Specimen	Able to Perform	Able to Perform with Assistance	Unable to Perform	Initials and Date
1. Carry out beginning procedure actions. *Comments:*	☐	☐	☐	
2. Assemble equipment. *Comments:*	☐	☐	☐	
3. Fill out the label on the specimen container. *Comments:*	☐	☐	☐	
4. Wash your hands. *Comments:*	☐	☐	☐	
5. Apply disposable gloves. *Comments:*	☐	☐	☐	
6. Offer the bedpan, instructing the patient not to place tissue in the pan. *Comments:*	☐	☐	☐	
7. After the patient voids, cover the pan and place on a protected chair. *Comments:*	☐	☐	☐	
8. Carefully pour about 120 mL of urine into a specimen container. *Comments:*	☐	☐	☐	
9. Remove and dispose of gloves. *Comments:*	☐	☐	☐	
10. If patient can ambulate, place a specimen collector in the toilet. *Comments:*	☐	☐	☐	

continued on the following page

continued from the previous page

Procedure 115	Able to Perform	Able to Perform with Assistance	Unable to Perform	Initials and Date
11. Assist the patient to the bathroom and instruct her not to place tissue in the collector. *Comments:*	☐	☐	☐	
12. Provide privacy while the patient voids. *Comments:*	☐	☐	☐	
13. When patient is finished, apply gloves. *Comments:*	☐	☐	☐	
14. Remove the specimen container and note the amount of urine if necessary. *Comments:*	☐	☐	☐	
15. Remove the cap and place it on a flat surface with the clean side facing up. *Comments:*	☐	☐	☐	
16. Carefully pour about 120 mL of urine into a specimen container. *Comments:*	☐	☐	☐	
17. Remove and dispose of gloves. *Comments:*	☐	☐	☐	
18. Wash your hands. *Comments:*	☐	☐	☐	
19. Place the cap on the specimen container. *Comments:*	☐	☐	☐	
20. Attach completed label to the container. *Comments:*	☐	☐	☐	
21. Place the specimen in a biohazard specimen transport bag and attach a laboratory requisition slip. *Comments:*	☐	☐	☐	
22. Carry out procedure completion actions. *Comments:*	☐	☐	☐	
23. Follow the policy for transporting the specimen to the laboratory. *Comments:*	☐	☐	☐	

Checklist for Procedure 116   Collecting a Clean-Catch Urine Specimen

Name _____ Date _____

School _____

Instructor _____

Course _____

Procedure 116 **Collecting a Clean-Catch Urine Specimen**	Able to Perform	Able to Perform with Assistance	Unable to Perform	Initials and Date
1. Carry out beginning procedure actions. *Comments:*	☐	☐	☐	
2. Assemble equipment. *Comments:*	☐	☐	☐	
3. Wash your hands. *Comments:*	☐	☐	☐	
4. Apply disposable gloves. *Comments:*	☐	☐	☐	
5. Wash the patient's genital area. If the area is soiled, perform perineal care. *Comments:*	☐	☐	☐	
6. Open the container and place the cap on a flat surface with the clean inside facing up. *Comments:*	☐	☐	☐	
7. Instruct the patient to void. *Comments:*	☐	☐	☐	
8. Allow the first part of the urine to escape; then catch the urine stream in the sterile specimen container. *Comments:*	☐	☐	☐	
9. Allow the last portion of the urine stream to escape. *Comments:*	☐	☐	☐	
10. Place the sterile cap on the urine container immediately. *Comments:*	☐	☐	☐	

continued on the following page

continued from the previous page

Procedure 116	Able to Perform	Able to Perform with Assistance	Unable to Perform	Initials and Date
11. Allow the patient to wash her hands. *Comments:*	☐	☐	☐	
12. Wash and dry the outside of the specimen container. *Comments:*	☐	☐	☐	
13. Remove and dispose of gloves. *Comments:*	☐	☐	☐	
14. Wash your hands. *Comments:*	☐	☐	☐	
15. Attach a completed label to the container. *Comments:*	☐	☐	☐	
16. Place the specimen in a biohazard specimen transport bag and attach a laboratory requisition slip. *Comments:*	☐	☐	☐	
17. Carry out procedure completion actions. *Comments:*	☐	☐	☐	
18. Follow the policy for transporting the specimen to the laboratory. *Comments:*	☐	☐	☐	

Checklist for Procedure 117   Collecting a 24-Hour Urine Specimen

Name _____ Date _____

School _____

Instructor _____

Course _____

Procedure 117 Collecting a 24-Hour Urine Specimen	Able to Perform	Able to Perform with Assistance	Unable to Perform	Initials and Date
1. Carry out beginning procedure actions. *Comments:*	☐	☐	☐	
2. Assemble equipment. *Comments:*	☐	☐	☐	
3. Label the 24-hour specimen container. *Comments:*	☐	☐	☐	
4. Emphasize to the patient the necessity of saving all urine passed. *Comments:*	☐	☐	☐	
5. Place specimen container in the bathroom in a pan of ice. *Comments:*	☐	☐	☐	
6. Apply disposable gloves. *Comments:*	☐	☐	☐	
7. Allow the patient to void. *Comments:*	☐	☐	☐	
8. Place a "Save all urine—24 hour specimen" sign on the patient's door. *Comments:*	☐	☐	☐	
9. Instruct the patient not to place tissue in the specimen collection container. *Comments:*	☐	☐	☐	
10. At the end of the 24-hour period, ask patient to void one last time and add it to the specimen container. *Comments:*	☐	☐	☐	

continued on the following page

continued from the previous page

Procedure 117	Able to Perform	Able to Perform with Assistance	Unable to Perform	Initials and Date
11. Apply disposable gloves. *Comments:*	☐	☐	☐	
12. Remove the sign from the patient's door. *Comments:*	☐	☐	☐	
13. Check the label and attach the appropriate requisition slip. *Comments:*	☐	☐	☐	
14. Remove and dispose of gloves. *Comments:*	☐	☐	☐	
15. Place specimen in a biohazard specimen transport bag. *Comments:*	☐	☐	☐	
16. Carry out procedure completion actions. *Comments:*	☐	☐	☐	
17. Clean and replace equipment. *Comments:*	☐	☐	☐	
18. Follow the policy for transporting the specimen to the laboratory. *Comments:*	☐	☐	☐	

Checklist for Procedure 118 Testing Urine with the HemaCombistix®

Name _____ Date _____

School _____

Instructor _____

Course _____

Procedure 118 Testing Urine with the HemaCombistix®	Able to Perform	Able to Perform with Assistance	Unable to Perform	Initials and Date
1. Assemble equipment. *Comments:*	☐	☐	☐	
2. Wash your hands and apply disposable gloves. *Comments:*	☐	☐	☐	
3. Take reagent strips and the urine sample to the bathroom. *Comments:*	☐	☐	☐	
4. Remove the cap and place it on the counter. *Comments:*	☐	☐	☐	
5. Remove one reagent strip. *Comments:*	☐	☐	☐	
6. Dip the reagent end of the strip into the urine and remove immediately. *Comments:*	☐	☐	☐	
7. Tap the edge of the strip to remove excess urine. *Comments:*	☐	☐	☐	
8. Compare the reagent side of the test area with the color chart on the bottle. *Comments:*	☐	☐	☐	
9. Remove and dispose of gloves. *Comments:*	☐	☐	☐	
10. Carry out procedure completion actions. *Comments:*	☐	☐	☐	

Checklist for Procedure 119   Routine Drainage Check

Name _____ Date _____

School _____

Instructor _____

Course _____

Procedure 119 Routine Drainage Check	Able to Perform	Able to Perform with Assistance	Unable to Perform	Initials and Date
1. Carry out beginning procedure actions. *Comments:*	☐	☐	☐	
2. Wash your hands and apply disposable gloves. *Comments:*	☐	☐	☐	
3. Raise the bedding and observe the tubing. *Comments:*	☐	☐	☐	
4. Check the condition of the catheter and the meatus. *Comments:*	☐	☐	☐	
5. Check that the drainage tubing is coiled on the bed. *Comments:*	☐	☐	☐	
6. Make sure that the collection bag is lower than the patient's hips. *Comments:*	☐	☐	☐	
7. Keep the end of the drainage tube above the urine level in the bag. *Comments:*	☐	☐	☐	
8. Be sure that the urine bag is attached to the bed frame. *Comments:*	☐	☐	☐	
9. Note the color, character, and flow of urine. *Comments:*	☐	☐	☐	
10. Measure the urine. *Comments:*	☐	☐	☐	
11. Remove and dispose of gloves. *Comments:*	☐	☐	☐	
12. Carry out procedure completion actions. *Comments:*	☐	☐	☐	

Checklist for Procedure 120   Giving Indwelling Catheter Care

Name _____ Date _____

School _____

Instructor _____

Course _____

Procedure 120 Giving Indwelling Catheter Care	Able to Perform	Able to Perform with Assistance	Unable to Perform	Initials and Date
1. Carry out beginning procedure actions. *Comments:*	☐	☐	☐	
2. Assemble equipment. *Comments:*	☐	☐	☐	
3. Raise the bed to a comfortable working height. *Comments:*	☐	☐	☐	
4. Raise the opposite side rail and secure. *Comments:*	☐	☐	☐	
5. Position the patient on his back, with legs separated and knees bent. *Comments:*	☐	☐	☐	
6. Cover the patient with a bath blanket. *Comments:*	☐	☐	☐	
7. Fanfold bedding to the foot of the bed. *Comments:*	☐	☐	☐	
8. Ask the patient to raise the hips. *Comments:*	☐	☐	☐	
9. Place a protector underneath the patient. *Comments:*	☐	☐	☐	
10. Arrange a catheter care kit on the overbed table. *Comments:*	☐	☐	☐	
11. Open the kit and position at the foot of the bed. *Comments:*	☐	☐	☐	

continued on the following page

continued from the previous page

Procedure 120	Able to Perform	Able to Perform with Assistance	Unable to Perform	Initials and Date
12. Wash your hands and apply disposable gloves. *Comments:*	☐	☐	☐	
13. Draw the bath blanket back to expose only the genitals. *Comments:*	☐	☐	☐	
14. For the male patient, gently grasp the penis and draw the foreskin back. *Comments:*	☐	☐	☐	
15. Use an applicator dipped in antiseptic solution to cleanse the glans from the meatus toward the shaft for approximately 4 inches. *Comments:*	☐	☐	☐	
16. Use a clean applicator for each stroke and dispose of the used one. *Comments:*	☐	☐	☐	
17. Return the foreskin to its proper position. *Comments:*	☐	☐	☐	
18. For the female patient, separate the labia. *Comments:*	☐	☐	☐	
19. Use an applicator dipped in antiseptic solution to cleanse from front to back. *Comments:*	☐	☐	☐	
20. Begin at the center, then cleanse each side. *Comments:*	☐	☐	☐	
21. Use a clean applicator for each stroke and dispose of the used one. *Comments:*	☐	☐	☐	
22. Clean the catheter down about 4 inches. *Comments:*	☐	☐	☐	
23. Dry carefully. *Comments:*	☐	☐	☐	

Procedure 120	Able to Perform	Able to Perform with Assistance	Unable to Perform	Initials and Date
24. Remove and dispose of gloves. *Comments:*	☐	☐	☐	
25. Wash your hands. *Comments:*	☐	☐	☐	
26. Check the security of the catheter. *Comments:*	☐	☐	☐	
27. Check to be assure that the tubing is coiled on the bed and that it hangs straight down. *Comments:*	☐	☐	☐	
28. Empty the bag and measure the contents, if necessary. *Comments:*	☐	☐	☐	
29. Replace bedding and remove the bath blanket. *Comments:*	☐	☐	☐	
30. Fold the bath blanket and store or place in linen hamper. *Comments:*	☐	☐	☐	
31. Lower the bed. *Comments:*	☐	☐	☐	
32. Adjust the side rails for safety. *Comments:*	☐	☐	☐	
33. Carry out procedure completion actions. *Comments:*	☐	☐	☐	

Checklist for Procedure 121 Emptying a Urinary Drainage Unit

Name _____ Date _____

School _____

Instructor _____

Course _____

Procedure 121 **Emptying a Urinary Drainage Unit**	Able to Perform	Able to Perform with Assistance	Unable to Perform	Initials and Date
1. Carry out beginning procedure actions. *Comments:*	☐	☐	☐	
2. Assemble equipment. *Comments:*	☐	☐	☐	
3. Wash your hands. *Comments:*	☐	☐	☐	
4. Apply disposable gloves. *Comments:*	☐	☐	☐	
5. Place a paper towel on the floor under the drainage bag. *Comments:*	☐	☐	☐	
6. Place a graduate on the paper towel under the drain of the collection bag. *Comments:*	☐	☐	☐	
7. Remove the drain from the holder, open, and allow urine to flow into the graduate. *Comments:*	☐	☐	☐	
8. Close the drain and replace it in the holder. *Comments:*	☐	☐	☐	
9. If contamination occurs, wipe the drain with an antiseptic wipe and dispose of the wipe. *Comments:*	☐	☐	☐	
10. Check the drainage tube position. *Comments:*	☐	☐	☐	

continued on the following page

continued from the previous page

Procedure 121	Able to Perform	Able to Perform with Assistance	Unable to Perform	Initials and Date
11. Pick up and discard the paper towel. *Comments:*	☐	☐	☐	
12. Empty the graduate in the bathroom. *Comments:*	☐	☐	☐	
13. Wash, dry, and store the graduate. *Comments:*	☐	☐	☐	
14. Record the amount of urine and note its character. *Comments:*	☐	☐	☐	
15. Remove and dispose of gloves. *Comments:*	☐	☐	☐	
16. Carry out procedure completion actions. *Comments:*	☐	☐	☐	

Checklist for Procedure 122   Disconnecting the Catheter

Name _____ Date _____

School _____

Instructor _____

Course _____

Procedure 122 **Disconnecting the Catheter**	Able to Perform	Able to Perform with Assistance	Unable to Perform	Initials and Date
1. Carry out beginning procedure actions. *Comments:*	☐	☐	☐	
2. Assemble equipment. *Comments:*	☐	☐	☐	
3. Wash your hands. *Comments:*	☐	☐	☐	
4. Apply disposable gloves. *Comments:*	☐	☐	☐	
5. Clamp the catheter. *Comments:*	☐	☐	☐	
6. Disconnect the catheter and drainage tubing. *Comments:*	☐	☐	☐	
7. If contamination occurs, wipe the drain with an antiseptic wipe and dispose of the wipe. *Comments:*	☐	☐	☐	
8. Insert a sterile plug in the end of the catheter. *Comments:*	☐	☐	☐	
9. Place a sterile cap over the exposed end of the drainage tube. *Comments:*	☐	☐	☐	
10. Secure the drainage tube to the bed frame. *Comments:*	☐	☐	☐	

continued on the following page

continued from the previous page

Procedure 122	Able to Perform	Able to Perform with Assistance	Unable to Perform	Initials and Date
11. Remove and dispose of gloves. *Comments:*	☐	☐	☐	
12. Wash your hands. *Comments:*	☐	☐	☐	
13. Carry out procedure completion actions. *Comments:*	☐	☐	☐	

Checklist for Procedure 123   Applying a Condom for Urinary Drainage

Name _____ Date _____

School _____

Instructor _____

Course _____

Procedure 123 Applying a Condom for Urinary Drainage	Able to Perform	Able to Perform with Assistance	Unable to Perform	Initials and Date
1. Carry out beginning procedure actions. *Comments:*	☐	☐	☐	
2. Assemble equipment. *Comments:*	☐	☐	☐	
3. Arrange equipment on the overbed table. *Comments:*	☐	☐	☐	
4. Raise the bed to a comfortable working height. *Comments:*	☐	☐	☐	
5. Raise and secure the opposite side rail. *Comments:*	☐	☐	☐	
6. Lower the side rail on the side you are working. *Comments:*	☐	☐	☐	
7. Cover the patient with a bath blanket. *Comments:*	☐	☐	☐	
8. Fanfold bedding to the foot of the bed. *Comments:*	☐	☐	☐	
9. Wash your hands. *Comments:*	☐	☐	☐	
10. Apply disposable gloves. *Comments:*	☐	☐	☐	
11. Place a bed protector under the patient's hips. *Comments:*	☐	☐	☐	

continued on the following page

continued from the previous page

Procedure 123	Able to Perform	Able to Perform with Assistance	Unable to Perform	Initials and Date
12. Expose the genitals. *Comments:*	☐	☐	☐	
13. Carefully wash and dry the penis. *Comments:*	☐	☐	☐	
14. Check the condom for "ready stick" surface. *Comments:*	☐	☐	☐	
15. Place the condom at the top of the penis and roll it toward the base. *Comments:*	☐	☐	☐	
16. Check to ensure that the foreskin is in normal position, if necessary. *Comments:*	☐	☐	☐	
17. Secure the condom to the penis. *Comments:*	☐	☐	☐	
18. Connect the condom to the drainage tubing on the collection bag. *Comments:*	☐	☐	☐	
19. Remove and dispose of gloves. *Comments:*	☐	☐	☐	
20. Wash your hands. *Comments:*	☐	☐	☐	
21. Adjust bedding and remove the bath blanket. *Comments:*	☐	☐	☐	
22. Fold the bath blanket and store or place in the linen hamper. *Comments:*	☐	☐	☐	
23. Lower the bed. *Comments:*	☐	☐	☐	

Procedure 123	Able to Perform	Able to Perform with Assistance	Unable to Perform	Initials and Date
24. Adjust the side rails for safety. *Comments:*	☐	☐	☐	
25. Carry out procedure completion actions. *Comments:*	☐	☐	☐	
26. Wash your hands. *Comments:*	☐	☐	☐	
27. To change the catheter, apply disposable gloves and remove the adhesive strip and roll the condom back over the tip of the penis. *Comments:*	☐	☐	☐	
28. Discard in a plastic bag. *Comments:*	☐	☐	☐	
29. Observe the skin for abnormalities and report any to the nurse. *Comments:*	☐	☐	☐	
30. Remove disposable gloves. *Comments:*	☐	☐	☐	
31. Wash your hands. *Comments:*	☐	☐	☐	

Checklist for Procedure 124   Connecting a Catheter to a Leg Bag

Name _____ Date _____

School _____

Instructor _____

Course _____

Procedure 124 Connecting a Catheter to a Leg Bag	Able to Perform	Able to Perform with Assistance	Unable to Perform	Initials and Date
1. Carry out beginning procedure actions. *Comments:*	☐	☐	☐	
2. Assemble equipment. *Comments:*	☐	☐	☐	
3. Wash your hands. *Comments:*	☐	☐	☐	
4. Apply disposable gloves. *Comments:*	☐	☐	☐	
5. Place a bed protector under the catheter and drainage tube connection. *Comments:*	☐	☐	☐	
6. Clamp the catheter. *Comments:*	☐	☐	☐	
7. Disconnect the catheter and drainage tube. *Comments:*	☐	☐	☐	
8. Insert a sterile plug in the end of the catheter. *Comments:*	☐	☐	☐	
9. Place a sterile cap over the exposed end of the drainage tube. *Comments:*	☐	☐	☐	
10. If contamination occurs, wipe the drain with an antiseptic wipe and dispose of the wipe. *Comments:*	☐	☐	☐	

continued on the following page

continued from the previous page

Procedure 124	Able to Perform	Able to Perform with Assistance	Unable to Perform	Initials and Date
11. Secure the drainage tube to the bed frame. *Comments:*	☐	☐	☐	
12. Remove the catheter plug. *Comments:*	☐	☐	☐	
13. Insert the end of the leg bag tubing into the catheter. *Comments:*	☐	☐	☐	
14. Release the catheter clamp. *Comments:*	☐	☐	☐	
15. Secure the leg bag to the patient's leg. *Comments:*	☐	☐	☐	
16. Check for correct placement of the tubing and leakage. *Comments:*	☐	☐	☐	
17. Remove the bed protector and discard it. *Comments:*	☐	☐	☐	
18. Remove and dispose of gloves. *Comments:*	☐	☐	☐	
19. Wash your hands. *Comments:*	☐	☐	☐	
20. Assist the patient out of bed. *Comments:*	☐	☐	☐	
21. Discard single use leg bag in a biohazardous waste container. *Comments:*	☐	☐	☐	
22. Carry out procedure completion actions. *Comments:*	☐	☐	☐	

Checklist for Procedure 125   Emptying a Leg Bag

Name _____ Date _____

School _____

Instructor _____

Course _____

Procedure 125 Emptying a Leg Bag	Able to Perform	Able to Perform with Assistance	Unable to Perform	Initials and Date
1. Carry out beginning procedure actions. *Comments:*	☐	☐	☐	
2. Assemble equipment. *Comments:*	☐	☐	☐	
3. Position the patient safely. *Comments:*	☐	☐	☐	
4. Wash your hands. *Comments:*	☐	☐	☐	
5. Apply disposable gloves. *Comments:*	☐	☐	☐	
6. Release the Velcro straps securing the bag to the patient's leg. *Comments:*	☐	☐	☐	
7. Place a paper towel on the floor under the drainage outlet of the leg bag. *Comments:*	☐	☐	☐	
8. Place a graduate on the paper towel under the drainage outlet. *Comments:*	☐	☐	☐	
9. Remove the cap. *Comments:*	☐	☐	☐	
10. Drain the collected urine into the graduate. *Comments:*	☐	☐	☐	

continued on the following page

continued from the previous page

Procedure 125	Able to Perform	Able to Perform with Assistance	Unable to Perform	Initials and Date
11. If contamination occurs, wipe the drain with an antiseptic wipe and dispose of the wipe. *Comments:*	☐	☐	☐	
12. Wipe the drainage outlet with an antiseptic wipe. *Comments:*	☐	☐	☐	
13. Replace the cap. *Comments:*	☐	☐	☐	
14. Refasten the leg bag to the patient's leg. *Comments:*	☐	☐	☐	
15. Make sure the patient is comfortable and safe. *Comments:*	☐	☐	☐	
16. Discard the paper towel. *Comments:*	☐	☐	☐	
17. Measure the urine and note the amount. *Comments:*	☐	☐	☐	
18. Discard the urine. *Comments:*	☐	☐	☐	
19. Clean and store the graduate. *Comments:*	☐	☐	☐	
20. Remove and dispose of gloves. *Comments:*	☐	☐	☐	
21. Carry out procedure completion actions. *Comments:*	☐	☐	☐	

Checklist for Procedure 126   Breast Self-Examination

Name _____ Date _____

School _____

Instructor _____

Course _____

Procedure 126 Breast Self-Examination	Able to Perform	Able to Perform with Assistance	Unable to Perform	Initials and Date
1. Disrobe above the waist. *Comments:*	☐	☐	☐	
2. Stand or sit in front of a mirror. *Comments:*	☐	☐	☐	
3. Observe breasts for changes in shape or size. *Comments:*	☐	☐	☐	
4. Raise your hands above your head and clasp hands. *Comments:*	☐	☐	☐	
5. Press inward with your hands while observing the breasts. *Comments:*	☐	☐	☐	
6. Note any dimpling of the breast tissue. *Comments:*	☐	☐	☐	
7. Fold a small towel. *Comments:*	☐	☐	☐	
8. Lie on a bed with a towel under your right shoulder. *Comments:*	☐	☐	☐	
9. Flex your right arm and bring it over your head. *Comments:*	☐	☐	☐	
10. Use the fingertips of your left hand to examine the right breast. *Comments:*	☐	☐	☐	

continued on the following page

continued from the previous page

Procedure 126	Able to Perform	Able to Perform with Assistance	Unable to Perform	Initials and Date
11. Using a rolling motion, start at the nipple and work around the entire breast so that all tissue is examined. *Comments:*	☐	☐	☐	
12. Examine the right axilla in the same way. *Comments:*	☐	☐	☐	
13. Repeat the procedure with the opposite breast and axilla. *Comments:*	☐	☐	☐	

Checklist for Procedure 127   Giving a Nonsterile Vaginal Douche

Name _____ Date _____

School _____

Instructor _____

Course _____

Procedure 127 **Giving a Nonsterile Vaginal Douche**	Able to Perform	Able to Perform with Assistance	Unable to Perform	Initials and Date
1. Carry out beginning procedure actions. *Comments:*	☐	☐	☐	
2. Assemble equipment. *Comments:*	☐	☐	☐	
3. Pour disinfecting solution over cotton balls. *Comments:*	☐	☐	☐	
4. Measure water into the douche container. *Comments:*	☐	☐	☐	
5. Add powder or solution as ordered. *Comments:*	☐	☐	☐	
6. Hang the douche bag on a standard. *Comments:*	☐	☐	☐	
7. Close the clamp on the tubing and leave the protector on the sterile tip. *Comments:*	☐	☐	☐	
8. Place a bed protector on a chair and assemble equipment within reach. *Comments:*	☐	☐	☐	
9. Screen the unit. *Comments:*	☐	☐	☐	
10. Elevate the bed to a comfortable working height and put up side rails for safety. *Comments:*	☐	☐	☐	

continued on the following page

continued from the previous page

Procedure 127	Able to Perform	Able to Perform with Assistance	Unable to Perform	Initials and Date
11. Wash your hands. *Comments:*	☐	☐	☐	
12. Apply disposable gloves. *Comments:*	☐	☐	☐	
13. Lower the side rail on the working side. *Comments:*	☐	☐	☐	
14. Assist the patient into the dorsal recumbent position. *Comments:*	☐	☐	☐	
15. Place a bed protector under the patient's buttocks. *Comments:*	☐	☐	☐	
16. Remove perineal pad from front to back and discard. *Comments:*	☐	☐	☐	
17. Drape the patient with a bed blanket. *Comments:*	☐	☐	☐	
18. Fanfold top bedding to the foot of the bed. *Comments:*	☐	☐	☐	
19. Place a bedpan under the patient and have her void. *Comments:*	☐	☐	☐	
20. If necessary, empty bedpan. *Comments:*	☐	☐	☐	
21. Cleanse the patient's perineum. *Comments:*	☐	☐	☐	
22. Replace the bedpan, if necessary. *Comments:*	☐	☐	☐	
23. Position the patient in the dorsal recumbent position and readjust the bed blanket. *Comments:*	☐	☐	☐	

continued from the previous page

Procedure 127	Able to Perform	Able to Perform with Assistance	Unable to Perform	Initials and Date
24. Elevate the head of the bed for comfort, if necessary. *Comments:*	☐	☐	☐	
25. Open the clamp to expel air. *Comments:*	☐	☐	☐	
26. Remove the protector from the sterile tip. *Comments:*	☐	☐	☐	
27. Allow a small amount of solution to flow over the inner thigh and over the vulva. *Comments:*	☐	☐	☐	
28. While the solution continues to flow, insert the nozzle slowly and gently with an upward and backward movement into the vagina for about 3 inches. *Comments:*	☐	☐	☐	
29. Rotate the nozzle from side to side. *Comments:*	☐	☐	☐	
30. When the douche is empty, remove the nozzle slowly and clamp the tubing. *Comments:*	☐	☐	☐	
31. Have the patient sit up on a bedpan. *Comments:*	☐	☐	☐	
32. Remove the douche bag from the standard and place it on the bed protector. *Comments:*	☐	☐	☐	
33. Dry the perineum with tissue and discard tissue in the bedpan. *Comments:*	☐	☐	☐	
34. Cover the bedpan and place it on the bed protector on the chair. *Comments:*	☐	☐	☐	
35. Have the patient turn on her side. *Comments:*	☐	☐	☐	

continued on the following page

continued from the previous page

Procedure 127	Able to Perform	Able to Perform with Assistance	Unable to Perform	Initials and Date
36. Dry the patient's buttocks with tissue. *Comments:*	☐	☐	☐	
37. Place a clean pad over the vulva from front to back. *Comments:*	☐	☐	☐	
38. Remove the bed protector and bath blanket. *Comments:*	☐	☐	☐	
39. Replace the top bedding. *Comments:*	☐	☐	☐	
40. Observe the contents of the bedpan and then discard the contents according to policy. *Comments:*	☐	☐	☐	
41. Follow policy for equipment care. *Comments:*	☐	☐	☐	
42. Remove and dispose of gloves. *Comments:*	☐	☐	☐	
43. Wash your hands. *Comments:*	☐	☐	☐	
44. Carry out procedure completion actions. *Comments:*	☐	☐	☐	

Checklist for Procedure 128   Changing a Diaper

Name _____ Date _____

School _____

Instructor _____

Course _____

Procedure 128 Changing a Diaper	Able to Perform	Able to Perform with Assistance	Unable to Perform	Initials and Date
1. Carry out beginning procedure actions. *Comments:*	☐	☐	☐	
2. Assemble equipment. *Comments:*	☐	☐	☐	
3. Apply disposable gloves. *Comments:*	☐	☐	☐	
4. Remove the soiled diaper. *Comments:*	☐	☐	☐	
5. Observe the stool color, consistency, and quality. *Comments:*	☐	☐	☐	
6. Roll the diaper so that the clean outer side faces out. *Comments:*	☐	☐	☐	
7. Place in the trash or out of reach of the infant. *Comments:*	☐	☐	☐	
8. Cleanse the diaper area. *Comments:*	☐	☐	☐	
9. Discard the wipes or washcloth. *Comments:*	☐	☐	☐	
10. Lift the buttocks with one hand. *Comments:*	☐	☐	☐	
11. Slide the new, open diaper under the infant. *Comments:*	☐	☐	☐	

continued on the following page

continued from the previous page

Procedure 128	Able to Perform	Able to Perform with Assistance	Unable to Perform	Initials and Date
12. Pull the diaper between the legs. *Comments:*	☐	☐	☐	
13. Fold the top edge of the diaper down and position under the umbilical cord. *Comments:*	☐	☐	☐	
14. Fasten the tape snugly on each side. *Comments:*	☐	☐	☐	
15. Perform cord care. *Comments:*	☐	☐	☐	
16. Change other clothing if necessary. *Comments:*	☐	☐	☐	
17. Discard the soiled diaper. *Comments:*	☐	☐	☐	
18. Remove and discard gloves. *Comments:*	☐	☐	☐	
19. Carry out procedure completion actions. *Comments:*	☐	☐	☐	

Checklist for Procedure 129   Bathing an Infant

Name _____ Date _____

School _____

Instructor _____

Course _____

Procedure 129 Bathing an Infant	Able to Perform	Able to Perform with Assistance	Unable to Perform	Initials and Date
1. Carry out beginning procedure actions. *Comments:*	☐	☐	☐	
2. Assemble equipment. *Comments:*	☐	☐	☐	
3. Place the infant in a bassinet with sides. *Comments:*	☐	☐	☐	
4. Place supplies within easy reach. *Comments:*	☐	☐	☐	
5. Check the infant's skin and report any abnormalities. *Comments:*	☐	☐	☐	
6. Check the umbilical card and report any abnormalities. *Comments:*	☐	☐	☐	
7. Remove the infant's clothing. *Comments:*	☐	☐	☐	
8. Cover the infant with a blanket. *Comments:*	☐	☐	☐	
9. Cleanse the eyes with a moist cotton ball. *Comments:*	☐	☐	☐	
10. Wash the external ears with a clean moist cotton ball or washcloth. *Comments:*	☐	☐	☐	
11. Wash the face and neck with plain water. *Comments:*	☐	☐	☐	

continued on the following page

continued from the previous page

Procedure 129	Able to Perform	Able to Perform with Assistance	Unable to Perform	Initials and Date
12. Pat dry with a towel. *Comments:*	☐	☐	☐	
13. Expose the upper body and cleanse. *Comments:*	☐	☐	☐	
14. Rinse and dry the upper body. *Comments:*	☐	☐	☐	
15. Cleanse the area around the umbilicus. *Comments:*	☐	☐	☐	
16. Rinse and pat dry. *Comments:*	☐	☐	☐	
17. Cover the upper body with the blanket. *Comments:*	☐	☐	☐	
18. Expose the lower body. *Comments:*	☐	☐	☐	
19. Wash the legs and outer buttocks. *Comments:*	☐	☐	☐	
20. Rinse well and pat dry. *Comments:*	☐	☐	☐	
21. Use a clean washcloth and cleanse the genitalia with plain water. *Comments:*	☐	☐	☐	
22. Rinse and pat dry. *Comments:*	☐	☐	☐	
23. Cleanse the anal area with soap, rinse, and pat dry. *Comments:*	☐	☐	☐	
24. Diaper the infant. *Comments:*	☐	☐	☐	

Procedure 129	Able to Perform	Able to Perform with Assistance	Unable to Perform	Initials and Date
25. Wrap in a blanket. *Comments:*	☐	☐	☐	
26. Pick up the infant using a football hold. *Comments:*	☐	☐	☐	
27. Hold the head over the basin. *Comments:*	☐	☐	☐	
28. Wet the scalp well with a washcloth and water. *Comments:*	☐	☐	☐	
29. Lather and gently wash the scalp. *Comments:*	☐	☐	☐	
30. Rinse the scalp and pat dry. *Comments:*	☐	☐	☐	
31. Comb the infant's hair, cover the head, and dress the infant. *Comments:*	☐	☐	☐	
32. Replace the damp blanket and sheets. *Comments:*	☐	☐	☐	
33. Carry out procedure completion actions. *Comments:*	☐	☐	☐	

Checklist for Procedure 130 Admitting a Pediatric Patient

Name _____ Date _____

School _____

Instructor _____

Course _____

Procedure 130 Admitting a Pediatric Patient	Able to Perform	Able to Perform with Assistance	Unable to Perform	Initials and Date
1. Introduce yourself to the child and his parents. *Comments:*	☐	☐	☐	
2. Show them to the child's room and familiarize them with the unit. *Comments:*	☐	☐	☐	
3. Explain what you will do. *Comments:*	☐	☐	☐	
4. Wash your hands. *Comments:*	☐	☐	☐	
5. Place an identification band on the child. *Comments:*	☐	☐	☐	
6. Dress the child in his own pajamas or hospital clothing. *Comments:*	☐	☐	☐	
7. Obtain the child's height and weight and record each. *Comments:*	☐	☐	☐	
8. Measure vital signs. *Comments:*	☐	☐	☐	
9. Obtain urine specimen. *Comments:*	☐	☐	☐	
10. Wash your hands. *Comments:*	☐	☐	☐	

continued on the following page

continued from the previous page

Procedure 130	Able to Perform	Able to Perform with Assistance	Unable to Perform	Initials and Date
11. Assist with the examination if necessary. *Comments:*	☐	☐	☐	
12. Explain rooming-in and visiting policies to the parents. *Comments:*	☐	☐	☐	
13. If necessary, stay with the child to provide comfort. *Comments:*	☐	☐	☐	

Checklist for Procedure 131   Weighing the Pediatric Patient

Name _____ Date _____

School _____

Instructor _____

Course _____

Procedure 131 Weighing the Pediatric Patient	Able to Perform	Able to Perform with Assistance	Unable to Perform	Initials and Date
1. Wash your hands. *Comments:*	☐	☐	☐	
2. Cover the scale with a small blanket and then balance the scale. *Comments:*	☐	☐	☐	
3. Check the infant's previous weight. *Comments:*	☐	☐	☐	
4. Check the identification band. *Comments:*	☐	☐	☐	
5. Remove the infant's diaper and shirt. *Comments:*	☐	☐	☐	
6. Place the infant on the scale. *Comments:*	☐	☐	☐	
7. Move the bar to the correct weight until the scale balances. *Comments:*	☐	☐	☐	
8. Return the infant to the crib. *Comments:*	☐	☐	☐	
9. Record the weight. *Comments:*	☐	☐	☐	
10. Remove the linen from the scale and place in the laundry hamper. *Comments:*	☐	☐	☐	

continued on the following page

continued from the previous page

Procedure 131	Able to Perform	Able to Perform with Assistance	Unable to Perform	Initials and Date
11. Properly store the scale. *Comments:*	☐	☐	☐	
12. Wash your hands. *Comments:*	☐	☐	☐	
13. Bring an upright scale to the bedside of a child who can stand. *Comments:*	☐	☐	☐	
14. Balance the scale. *Comments:*	☐	☐	☐	
15. Wash your hands. *Comments:*	☐	☐	☐	
16. Check the identification band. *Comments:*	☐	☐	☐	
17. Check the child's previous weight. *Comments:*	☐	☐	☐	
18. Have the child stand on the scale in as few clothes as possible. *Comments:*	☐	☐	☐	
19. Move the bar to the correct weight until the scale balances. *Comments:*	☐	☐	☐	
20. Record the weight. *Comments:*	☐	☐	☐	
21. Return the child to bed. *Comments:*	☐	☐	☐	
22. Properly store the scale. *Comments:*	☐	☐	☐	
23. Wash your hands. *Comments:*	☐	☐	☐	

continued from the previous page

Checklist for Procedure 132   Changing Crib Linens

Name _____ Date _____

School _____

Instructor _____

Course _____

Procedure 132 Changing Crib Linens	Able to Perform	Able to Perform with Assistance	Unable to Perform	Initials and Date
1. Wash your hands. *Comments:*	☐	☐	☐	
2. Gather supplies. *Comments:*	☐	☐	☐	
3. Bathe the infant; diaper and dress her. *Comments:*	☐	☐	☐	
4. Place the infant in a safe place. *Comments:*	☐	☐	☐	
5. Apply disposable gloves if the linen is soiled. *Comments:*	☐	☐	☐	
6. Strip the linen from the crib and dispose it of according to policy. *Comments:*	☐	☐	☐	
7. Remove and dispose of gloves. *Comments:*	☐	☐	☐	
8. Wash your hands. *Comments:*	☐	☐	☐	
9. Place a clean sheet hem side down on the bed. *Comments:*	☐	☐	☐	
10. Make one side of the crib, miter the corners, and tuck in the side. *Comments:*	☐	☐	☐	

continued on the following page

continued from the previous page

Procedure 132	Able to Perform	Able to Perform with Assistance	Unable to Perform	Initials and Date
11. Pull down the crib top and pull up the crib side. *Comments:*	☐	☐	☐	
12. Make the opposite side of the crib, miter the corners, and tuck in the side. *Comments:*	☐	☐	☐	
13. Place a diaper pad on the top of the sheet. *Comments:*	☐	☐	☐	
14. Place a clean blanket at the bottom of the bed. *Comments:*	☐	☐	☐	
15. Arrange bumper pads around the sides of the crib. *Comments:*	☐	☐	☐	
16. Wash your hands. *Comments:*	☐	☐	☐	
17. Return the infant to the crib, cover with the blanket, and pull up the crib side. *Comments:*	☐	☐	☐	

Checklist for Procedure 133   Changing Crib Linens (Infant in Crib)

Name _____ Date _____

School _____

Instructor _____

Course _____

Procedure 133 Changing Crib Linens (Infant in Crib)	Able to Perform	Able to Perform with Assistance	Unable to Perform	Initials and Date
1. Wash your hands. *Comments:*	☐	☐	☐	
2. Gather linens. *Comments:*	☐	☐	☐	
3. Bathe, diaper, and dress the infant. *Comments:*	☐	☐	☐	
4. Pick up the infant and hold with one arm. *Comments:*	☐	☐	☐	
5. Strip off the old linen with your free hand. *Comments:*	☐	☐	☐	
6. Place a clean sheet hem side down on the bed. *Comments:*	☐	☐	☐	
7. Place the infant on the sheet. *Comments:*	☐	☐	☐	
8. Keep one hand on the infant at all times. *Comments:*	☐	☐	☐	
9. Make one side of the crib, miter the corners, and tuck in the side. *Comments:*	☐	☐	☐	
10. Remove your hand from the infant and pull up the crib side. *Comments:*	☐	☐	☐	

continued on the following page

continued from the previous page

Procedure 133	Able to Perform	Able to Perform with Assistance	Unable to Perform	Initials and Date
11. Go to the opposite side of the crib, let down the crib side, and place one hand on the infant. *Comments:*	☐	☐	☐	
12. Make the opposite side of the crib, miter the corners, and tuck in the side. *Comments:*	☐	☐	☐	
13. Place a diaper pad under the infant. *Comments:*	☐	☐	☐	
14. Cover the infant with a blanket if necessary. *Comments:*	☐	☐	☐	
15. Arrange bumper pads around the sides of the crib. *Comments:*	☐	☐	☐	
16. Pull up the crib side. *Comments:*	☐	☐	☐	
17. Wash your hands. *Comments:*	☐	☐	☐	

Checklist for Procedure 134   Measuring Pediatric Temperature

Name _____ Date _____

School _____

Instructor _____

Course _____

Procedure 134 **Measuring Pediatric Temperature**	Able to Perform	Able to Perform with Assistance	Unable to Perform	Initials and Date
Rectal Temperature				
1. Wash your hands. *Comments:*	☐	☐	☐	
2. Apply disposable gloves. *Comments:*	☐	☐	☐	
3. Check the identification band. *Comments:*	☐	☐	☐	
4. Explain the procedure to the parents and the child. *Comments:*	☐	☐	☐	
5. Inspect the thermometer. *Comments:*	☐	☐	☐	
6. Shake down the thermometer. *Comments:*	☐	☐	☐	
7. Cover the thermometer with a disposable sheath. *Comments:*	☐	☐	☐	
8. Lubricate the thermometer sheath. *Comments:*	☐	☐	☐	
9. Lay the child on his back on bed or on stomach across your lap. *Comments:*	☐	☐	☐	
10. Insert the thermometer $\frac{1}{2}$ inch into the rectum and hold securely. *Comments:*	☐	☐	☐	

continued on the following page

continued from the previous page

Procedure 134	Able to Perform	Able to Perform with Assistance	Unable to Perform	Initials and Date
11. Leave in place for 3 to 5 minutes. *Comments:*	☐	☐	☐	
12. Remove and discard the sheath. *Comments:*	☐	☐	☐	
13. Read the thermometer. *Comments:*	☐	☐	☐	
14. Remove and discard gloves. *Comments:*	☐	☐	☐	
15. Wash your hands. *Comments:*	☐	☐	☐	
16. Record the temperature. *Comments:*	☐	☐	☐	
17. Report any deviations according to policy. *Comments:*	☐	☐	☐	
Oral Temperature				
1. Wash your hands. *Comments:*	☐	☐	☐	
2. Apply disposable gloves. *Comments:*	☐	☐	☐	
3. Check the identification band. *Comments:*	☐	☐	☐	
4. Explain the procedure to the parents and the child. *Comments:*	☐	☐	☐	
5. Inspect the thermometer. *Comments:*	☐	☐	☐	

Procedure 134	Able to Perform	Able to Perform with Assistance	Unable to Perform	Initials and Date
6. Shake down the thermometer. *Comments:*	☐	☐	☐	
7. Cover the thermometer with a disposable sheath. *Comments:*	☐	☐	☐	
8. Instruct the child to hold the thermometer under her tongue. *Comments:*	☐	☐	☐	
9. Leave in place for 5 to 8 minutes. *Comments:*	☐	☐	☐	
10. Remove and discard the sheath. *Comments:*	☐	☐	☐	
11. Read the thermometer. *Comments:*	☐	☐	☐	
12. Remove and discard gloves. *Comments:*	☐	☐	☐	
13. Wash your hands. *Comments:*	☐	☐	☐	
14. Record the temperature. *Comments:*	☐	☐	☐	
15. Report any deviations according to policy. *Comments:*	☐	☐	☐	

continued on the following page

continued from the previous page

Procedure 134	Able to Perform	Able to Perform with Assistance	Unable to Perform	Initials and Date
Axillary Temperature				
1. Explain the procedure to the parents and the child. *Comments:*	☐	☐	☐	
2. Check the identification band. *Comments:*	☐	☐	☐	
3. Wash your hands. *Comments:*	☐	☐	☐	
4. Inspect the thermometer. *Comments:*	☐	☐	☐	
5. Shake down the thermometer. *Comments:*	☐	☐	☐	
6. Cover the thermometer with a disposable sheath. *Comments:*	☐	☐	☐	
7. Hold the child's arm close to the chest for 10 minutes. *Comments:*	☐	☐	☐	
8. Remove and discard the sheath. *Comments:*	☐	☐	☐	
9. Read the thermometer. *Comments:*	☐	☐	☐	
10. Wash your hands. *Comments:*	☐	☐	☐	
11. Record the temperature. *Comments:*	☐	☐	☐	
12. Report any deviations according to policy. *Comments:*	☐	☐	☐	

Procedure 134	Able to Perform	Able to Perform with Assistance	Unable to Perform	Initials and Date
Tympanic Temperature				
1. Explain the procedure to the parents and the child. *Comments:*	☐	☐	☐	
2. Check the identification band. *Comments:*	☐	☐	☐	
3. Wash your hands. *Comments:*	☐	☐	☐	
4. Check the lens on the thermometer. *Comments:*	☐	☐	☐	
5. Set appropriate mode. *Comments:*	☐	☐	☐	
6. Place a clean probe cover on probe. *Comments:*	☐	☐	☐	
7. Position the patient for access to the ear you will be using. *Comments:*	☐	☐	☐	
8. Position the ear according to age and fit the probe snugly into the ear. *Comments:*	☐	☐	☐	
9. Insert the probe at least one-third of the way into the ear canal, making sure it forms a complete seal. *Comments:*	☐	☐	☐	
10. Press the activation button. *Comments:*	☐	☐	☐	
11. Leave it in place until the display blinks or signals that the temperature is final. *Comments:*	☐	☐	☐	
12. Remove and discard the probe cover. *Comments:*	☐	☐	☐	

continued on the following page

continued from the previous page

Procedure 134	Able to Perform	Able to Perform with Assistance	Unable to Perform	Initials and Date
13. Wash your hands. *Comments:*	☐	☐	☐	
14. Record the temperature. *Comments:*	☐	☐	☐	
15. Report any deviations according to policy. *Comments:*	☐	☐	☐	

Checklist for Procedure 135   Determining Pediatric Heart Rate (Pulse)

Name _____ Date _____

School _____

Instructor _____

Course _____

Procedure 135 Determining Pediatric Heart Rate (Pulse)	Able to Perform	Able to Perform with Assistance	Unable to Perform	Initials and Date
1. Wash your hands. *Comments:*	☐	☐	☐	
2. Check the identification band. *Comments:*	☐	☐	☐	
3. Explain the procedure to the parents and the child. *Comments:*	☐	☐	☐	
4. Clean and dry the stethoscope earpieces and diaphragm. *Comments:*	☐	☐	☐	
5. Warm the diaphragm of the stethoscope. *Comments:*	☐	☐	☐	
6. Place the stethoscope over the patient's heart. *Comments:*	☐	☐	☐	
7. Count the number of beats you hear in a minute. *Comments:*	☐	☐	☐	
8. Clean and dry the stethoscope earpieces and diaphragm. *Comments:*	☐	☐	☐	
9. Wash your hands. *Comments:*	☐	☐	☐	
10. Record the results. *Comments:*	☐	☐	☐	
11. Report any deviations according to policy. *Comments:*	☐	☐	☐	

Checklist for Procedure 136   Counting Respiratory Rate

Name _____ Date _____

School _____

Instructor _____

Course _____

Procedure 136 Counting Respiratory Rate	Able to Perform	Able to Perform with Assistance	Unable to Perform	Initials and Date
1. In infants and toddlers, observe the abdominal muscles for breathing. *Comments:*	☐	☐	☐	
2. Count the respiratory rate for a minute. *Comments:*	☐	☐	☐	
3. In preschoolers and older children, leave fingers in place after counting the pulse. *Comments:*	☐	☐	☐	
4. Observe the chest and count the respiratory rate for one minute. *Comments:*	☐	☐	☐	
5. Note the depth and regularity of respirations. *Comments:*	☐	☐	☐	
6. Record the rate, depth, and regularity. *Comments:*	☐	☐	☐	

Checklist for Procedure 137 Measuring Pediatric Blood Pressure

Name _____ Date _____

School _____

Instructor _____

Course _____

Procedure 137 Measuring Pediatric Blood Pressure	Able to Perform	Able to Perform with Assistance	Unable to Perform	Initials and Date
1. Select the correct cuff size. *Comments:*	☐	☐	☐	
2. Assemble equipment. *Comments:*	☐	☐	☐	
3. Clean and dry the stethoscope earpieces and diaphragm. *Comments:*	☐	☐	☐	
4. Wash your hands. *Comments:*	☐	☐	☐	
5. Check the identification band. *Comments:*	☐	☐	☐	
6. Explain the procedure to the child (and parents, if present). *Comments:*	☐	☐	☐	
7. Wrap the cuff securely around the upper arm. *Comments:*	☐	☐	☐	
8. Feel for brachial pulse. *Comments:*	☐	☐	☐	
9. Place the stethoscope earpieces in your ears and the diaphragm near the pulse point. *Comments:*	☐	☐	☐	
10. Pump up the cuff until you no longer hear the pulse. *Comments:*	☐	☐	☐	

continued on the following page

continued from the previous page

Procedure 137	Able to Perform	Able to Perform with Assistance	Unable to Perform	Initials and Date
11. Release the valve and listen for systolic and diastolic sounds. *Comments:*	☐	☐	☐	
12. Wash your hands. *Comments:*	☐	☐	☐	
13. Record the results. *Comments:*	☐	☐	☐	

Checklist for Procedure 138   Bottle-Feeding an Infant

Name _____ Date _____

School _____

Instructor _____

Course _____

Procedure 138 Bottle-Feeding an Infant	Able to Perform	Able to Perform with Assistance	Unable to Perform	Initials and Date
1. Wash your hands. *Comments:*	☐	☐	☐	
2. Gather supplies. *Comments:*	☐	☐	☐	
3. Check the identification. *Comments:*	☐	☐	☐	
4. Pick up the infant. *Comments:*	☐	☐	☐	
5. Sit in a chair or rocker. *Comments:*	☐	☐	☐	
6. Hold the infant in the crook of your arm with the infant's head slightly raised. *Comments:*	☐	☐	☐	
7. Place a bib under the chin, covering the chest. *Comments:*	☐	☐	☐	
8. Tip the bottle so the nipple is filled with formula. *Comments:*	☐	☐	☐	
9. Stroke the infant's cheek closest to you and place the nipple in her mouth. *Comments:*	☐	☐	☐	
10. If the infant does not suck on the nipple, gently lift up under her chin to close her mouth on the nipple. *Comments:*	☐	☐	☐	

continued on the following page

continued from the previous page

Procedure 138	Able to Perform	Able to Perform with Assistance	Unable to Perform	Initials and Date
11. Hold the bottle so the nipple stays filled with formula. *Comments:*	☐	☐	☐	
12. Feed the ordered amount of formula and burp according to age. *Comments:*	☐	☐	☐	
13. If the infant vomits, remove the bottle, turn the infant to the side, and lower her head. *Comments:*	☐	☐	☐	
14. After feeding, return her to the crib and place her on her back or side. *Comments:*	☐	☐	☐	
15. Pull up the crib side. *Comments:*	☐	☐	☐	
16. Wash your hands. *Comments:*	☐	☐	☐	
17. Record the amount of formula taken. *Comments:*	☐	☐	☐	

Checklist for Procedure 139   Burping (Method A)

Name _____ Date _____

School _____

Instructor _____

Course _____

Procedure 139 Burping (Method A)	Able to Perform	Able to Perform with Assistance	Unable to Perform	Initials and Date
1. Place a diaper or cloth over your shoulder. *Comments:*	☐	☐	☐	
2. Lift the infant up to your shoulder, holding him close to your chest. *Comments:*	☐	☐	☐	
3. Hold the infant in place with one hand and use the other to gently rub the infant's back until he burps. *Comments:*	☐	☐	☐	

Checklist for Procedure 140 Burping (Method B)

Name _____ Date _____

School _____

Instructor _____

Course _____

Procedure 140 Burping (Method B)	Able to Perform	Able to Perform with Assistance	Unable to Perform	Initials and Date
1. Place a diaper or cloth under the infant's chin. *Comments:*	☐	☐	☐	
2. Place the child in a sitting or upright position. *Comments:*	☐	☐	☐	
3. Place one hand on the infant's chest to support the infant's weight. *Comments:*	☐	☐	☐	
4. With the other hand gently rub or pat the infant's back until he burps. *Comments:*	☐	☐	☐	

Checklist for Procedure 141   Testing for Occult Blood using Hemoccult® and Developer

Name _____ Date _____

School _____

Instructor _____

Course _____

Procedure 141 Testing for Occult Blood using Hemoccult® and Developer	Able to Perform	Able to Perform with Assistance	Unable to Perform	Initials and Date
1. Wash your hands. *Comments:*	☐	☐	☐	
2. Assemble equipment. *Comments:*	☐	☐	☐	
3. Place a paper towel on a flat surface. *Comments:*	☐	☐	☐	
4. Open the flap of the Hemoccult® packet to expose the guaiac paper. *Comments:*	☐	☐	☐	
5. Apply disposable gloves. *Comments:*	☐	☐	☐	
6. Use a tongue blade to take a small amount of feces and smear it on the area of the card marked A. *Comments:*	☐	☐	☐	
7. Repeat the procedure with fecal matter from a different part of the specimen and make a smear on the area marked B. *Comments:*	☐	☐	☐	
8. Close the tab and turn the packet over. *Comments:*	☐	☐	☐	
9. Open the back tab. *Comments:*	☐	☐	☐	
10. Apply two drops of Hemoccult® developer on the exposed guaiac paper. *Comments:*	☐	☐	☐	

continued on the following page

continued from the previous page

Procedure 141	Able to Perform	Able to Perform with Assistance	Unable to Perform	Initials and Date
11. Time the reaction. *Comments:*	☐	☐	☐	
12. Read the results 30 to 60 seconds later. *Comments:*	☐	☐	☐	
13. Check for the presence of blood in the smear. *Comments:*	☐	☐	☐	
14. Dispose of the specimen. *Comments:*	☐	☐	☐	
15. Clean the bedpan and dispose of the paper towel, packet, and tongue blade. *Comments:*	☐	☐	☐	
16. Remove and dispose of gloves. *Comments:*	☐	☐	☐	

Checklist for Procedure 142 Collecting a Urine Specimen through a Drainage Port

Name _____ Date _____

School _____

Instructor _____

Course _____

Procedure 142 **Collecting a Urine Specimen through a Drainage Port**	Able to Perform	Able to Perform with Assistance	Unable to Perform	Initials and Date
1. Carry out beginning procedure actions. *Comments:*	☐	☐	☐	
2. Assemble equipment. *Comments:*	☐	☐	☐	
3. Clamp the drainage tube half an hour before the sample is to be collected. *Comments:*	☐	☐	☐	
4. Wash your hands. *Comments:*	☐	☐	☐	
5. Return to the bedside after 30 minutes and apply disposable gloves. *Comments:*	☐	☐	☐	
6. Place a bed protector on the bed. *Comments:*	☐	☐	☐	
7. Put an emesis basin on the bed protector under the catheter drainage port. *Comments:*	☐	☐	☐	
8. Wipe the drainage port with an alcohol wipe and discard. *Comments:*	☐	☐	☐	
9. Carefully remove the cap on the syringe. *Comments:*	☐	☐	☐	
10. Attach the needle carefully. *Comments:*	☐	☐	☐	
11. Open the specimen container package. *Comments:*	☐	☐	☐	

continued on the following page

continued from the previous page

Procedure 142	Able to Perform	Able to Perform with Assistance	Unable to Perform	Initials and Date
12. Remove the lid and lay it on the bedside stand. *Comments:*	☐	☐	☐	
13. Insert the needle into the port and withdraw the specimen. *Comments:*	☐	☐	☐	
14. Carefully withdraw the needle. *Comments:*	☐	☐	☐	
15. Wipe the port with an alcohol wipe and discard. *Comments:*	☐	☐	☐	
16. Transfer the urine sample to the specimen container. *Comments:*	☐	☐	☐	
17. Cover the container. *Comments:*	☐	☐	☐	
18. Discard the needle and syringe into a sharps container. *Comments:*	☐	☐	☐	
19. Remove and dispose of gloves. *Comments:*	☐	☐	☐	
20. Wash your hands. *Comments:*	☐	☐	☐	
21. Remove the catheter clamp. *Comments:*	☐	☐	☐	
22. Complete the label and place the label on the container. *Comments:*	☐	☐	☐	
23. Place the specimen container in a biohazard specimen transport bag. *Comments:*	☐	☐	☐	
24. Attach the completed laboratory requisition. *Comments:*	☐	☐	☐	
25. Carry out procedure completion actions. *Comments:*	☐	☐	☐	
26. Transport according to policy. *Comments:*	☐	☐	☐	

Checklist for Procedure 143   Removing an Indwelling Catheter

Name _____ Date _____

School _____

Instructor _____

Course _____

Procedure 143 Removing an Indwelling Catheter	Able to Perform	Able to Perform with Assistance	Unable to Perform	Initials and Date
1. Carry out beginning procedure actions. *Comments:*	☐	☐	☐	
2. Assemble equipment. *Comments:*	☐	☐	☐	
3. Position an underpad under the patient's buttocks. *Comments:*	☐	☐	☐	
4. Remove the tape or Velcro strap securing the catheter to the leg. *Comments:*	☐	☐	☐	
5. Empty urine in the tubing into the drainage bag. *Comments:*	☐	☐	☐	
6. Open the syringe and attach to the inflation port. *Comments:*	☐	☐	☐	
7. Allow the inflation balloon to deflate into the syringe on its own. *Comments:*	☐	☐	☐	
8. When the balloon is empty, grasp the catheter close to the perineum. *Comments:*	☐	☐	☐	
9. Gently pull the catheter, stopping if you feel resistance. *Comments:*	☐	☐	☐	
10. Withdraw the catheter. *Comments:*	☐	☐	☐	

continued on the following page

continued from the previous page

Procedure 143	Able to Perform	Able to Perform with Assistance	Unable to Perform	Initials and Date
11. Disconnect the catheter from the drainage tubing. *Comments:*	☐	☐	☐	
12. Discard the catheter according to policy. *Comments:*	☐	☐	☐	
13. Remove and dispose of gloves. *Comments:*	☐	☐	☐	
14. Wash your hands. *Comments:*	☐	☐	☐	
15. Apply disposable gloves. *Comments:*	☐	☐	☐	
16. Perform perineal care. *Comments:*	☐	☐	☐	
17. Empty the catheter bag and measure the output. *Comments:*	☐	☐	☐	
18. Discard the empty bag according to policy. *Comments:*	☐	☐	☐	
19. Offer the bedpan, urinal, or take the patient to the bathroom in 2 to 4 hours. *Comments:*	☐	☐	☐	
20. Carry out procedure completion actions. *Comments:*	☐	☐	☐	

Checklist for Procedure 144   Giving Routine Stoma Care (Colostomy)

Name _____ Date _____

School _____

Instructor _____

Course _____

Procedure 144 Giving Routine Stoma Care (Colostomy)	Able to Perform	Able to Perform with Assistance	Unable to Perform	Initials and Date
1. Carry out beginning procedure actions. *Comments:*	☐	☐	☐	
2. Assemble equipment. *Comments:*	☐	☐	☐	
3. Place a bath blanket over the patient. *Comments:*	☐	☐	☐	
4. Fanfold the top bedding to the foot of the bed. *Comments:*	☐	☐	☐	
5. Wash your hands. *Comments:*	☐	☐	☐	
6. Apply disposable gloves. *Comments:*	☐	☐	☐	
7. Place a bed protector under the patient's hips. *Comments:*	☐	☐	☐	
8. Place a bedpan on a covered chair. *Comments:*	☐	☐	☐	
9. Remove the soiled disposable stoma bag. *Comments:*	☐	☐	☐	
10. Place the bag in a bedpan or plastic bag. *Comments:*	☐	☐	☐	
11. Note the amount and type of drainage. *Comments:*	☐	☐	☐	
12. Remove the belt holding the stoma bag and save it, if clean. *Comments:*	☐	☐	☐	

continued on the following page

continued from the previous page

Procedure 144	Able to Perform	Able to Perform with Assistance	Unable to Perform	Initials and Date
13. Remove feces and drainage around the stoma. *Comments:*	☐	☐	☐	
14. Wash, rinse, and dry the area around the stoma. *Comments:*	☐	☐	☐	
15. Apply barrier cream lightly around the stoma, if ordered. *Comments:*	☐	☐	☐	
16. Position a clean belt around the patient. *Comments:*	☐	☐	☐	
17. Check the stoma size to make sure the correct size barrier is used. *Comments:*	☐	☐	☐	
18. Apply a new barrier adhesive wafer around the stoma. *Comments:*	☐	☐	☐	
19. Place a clean ostomy bag over the stoma and secure the belt. *Comments:*	☐	☐	☐	
20. Remove the bed protector. *Comments:*	☐	☐	☐	
21. Change the bedding if necessary. *Comments:*	☐	☐	☐	
22. Remove and discard gloves. *Comments:*	☐	☐	☐	
23. Remove the bath blanket and replace the top bedding. *Comments:*	☐	☐	☐	
24. Dispose of used materials according to policy. *Comments:*	☐	☐	☐	
25. Empty, wash, dry, and store the bedpan. *Comments:*	☐	☐	☐	
26. Carry out procedure completion actions. *Comments:*	☐	☐	☐	

continued from the previous page

Checklist for Procedure 145   Routine Care of an Ileostomy (With Patient in Bed)

Name _____ Date _____

School _____

Instructor _____

Course _____

Procedure 145 **Routine Care of an Ileostomy** **(With Patient in Bed)**	Able to Perform	Able to Perform with Assistance	Unable to Perform	Initials and Date
1. Carry out beginning procedure actions. *Comments:*	☐	☐	☐	
2. Assemble equipment. *Comments:*	☐	☐	☐	
3. Raise the opposite side rail. *Comments:*	☐	☐	☐	
4. Elevate the head of the bed and assist the patient to turn on the side toward you. *Comments:*	☐	☐	☐	
5. Replace bedding with a bath blanket. *Comments:*	☐	☐	☐	
6. Wash your hands. *Comments:*	☐	☐	☐	
7. Apply disposable gloves. *Comments:*	☐	☐	☐	
8. Place a bed protector under the patient. *Comments:*	☐	☐	☐	
9. Place a bedpan on the protector against the patient. *Comments:*	☐	☐	☐	
10. Place the end of the ileostomy bag in the bedpan. *Comments:*	☐	☐	☐	

continued on the following page

continued from the previous page

Procedure 145	Able to Perform	Able to Perform with Assistance	Unable to Perform	Initials and Date
11. Open the clamp and allow the bag to drain. *Comments:*	☐	☐	☐	
12. Note the amount and character of drainage. *Comments:*	☐	☐	☐	
13. Wipe the end of the drainage sheath and move it out of the drainage. *Comments:*	☐	☐	☐	
14. Cover the bedpan. *Comments:*	☐	☐	☐	
15. Disconnect the belt from the appliance and remove the belt from the patient. *Comments:*	☐	☐	☐	
16. Apply a small amount of solvent around the ring of the appliance to loosen it and remove. *Comments:*	☐	☐	☐	
17. Cover the stoma with gauze. *Comments:*	☐	☐	☐	
18. Inspect the skin around the stoma. *Comments:*	☐	☐	☐	
19. Remove and dispose of the gauze. *Comments:*	☐	☐	☐	
20. Apply the ring or strip around the stoma. *Comments:*	☐	☐	☐	
21. Clamp the appliance bag and apply to the ring. *Comments:*	☐	☐	☐	
22. Remove and dispose of gloves. *Comments:*	☐	☐	☐	

Procedure 145	Able to Perform	Able to Perform with Assistance	Unable to Perform	Initials and Date
23. Adjust a clean belt in position around the patient and connect it to the appliance. *Comments:*	☐	☐	☐	
24. Remove the bath blanket. *Comments:*	☐	☐	☐	
25. Assist the patient to wash his hands. *Comments:*	☐	☐	☐	
26. Wash your hands. *Comments:*	☐	☐	☐	
27. Apply disposable gloves. *Comments:*	☐	☐	☐	
28. If reusable, wash the belt and allow it to dry. *Comments:*	☐	☐	☐	
29. Carry out procedure completion actions. *Comments:*	☐	☐	☐	

Checklist for Procedure 146   Setting up a Sterile Field using a Sterile Drape

Name _____ Date _____

School _____

Instructor _____

Course _____

Procedure 146 Setting up a Sterile Field using a Sterile Drape	Able to Perform	Able to Perform with Assistance	Unable to Perform	Initials and Date
1. Wash your hands. *Comments:*	☐	☐	☐	
2. Open the sterile package containing the sterile drape. *Comments:*	☐	☐	☐	
3. Use the thumb and index finger of your dominant hand to grasp the folded top edge of the drape. *Comments:*	☐	☐	☐	
4. Lift the drape out of the package. *Comments:*	☐	☐	☐	
5. Hold the drape away from your body and allow it to unfold. *Comments:*	☐	☐	☐	
6. Pick up the top corner on the other side of the drape after it unfolds. *Comments:*	☐	☐	☐	
7. Begin with the side opposite your body and slowly lay the drape across the table. *Comments:*	☐	☐	☐	
8. Open the other packages and add necessary equipment to the sterile field. *Comments:*	☐	☐	☐	

Checklist for Procedure 147   Adding an Item to a Sterile Field

Name _____ Date _____

School _____

Instructor _____

Course _____

Procedure 147 Adding an Item to a Sterile Field	Able to Perform	Able to Perform with Assistance	Unable to Perform	Initials and Date
1. Wash your hands. *Comments:*	☐	☐	☐	
2. Open the sterile package. *Comments:*	☐	☐	☐	
3. Grasp the package from the bottom. *Comments:*	☐	☐	☐	
4. Use your free hand to pull the sides of the package away from the sterile field. *Comments:*	☐	☐	☐	
5. If using a peel-away package, peel the sides apart and drop the inner package onto the sterile field. *Comments:*	☐	☐	☐	
6. Drop the sterile item onto the sterile field. *Comments:*	☐	☐	☐	
7. Discard the wrapper. *Comments:*	☐	☐	☐	

Checklist for Procedure 148 Adding Liquids to a Sterile Field

Name _____ Date _____

School _____

Instructor _____

Course _____

Procedure 148 Adding Liquids to a Sterile Field	Able to Perform	Able to Perform with Assistance	Unable to Perform	Initials and Date
1. Wash your hands. Comments:	☐	☐	☐	
2. Inspect the container. Comments:	☐	☐	☐	
3. Open the container of liquid. Comments:	☐	☐	☐	
4. Place the cap upright on a table. Comments:	☐	☐	☐	
5. Pour a small amount of solution into the sink or trashcan. Comments:	☐	☐	☐	
6. Hold the bottle at an angle 6 to 8 inches above a sterile bowl or container. Comments:	☐	☐	☐	
7. Slowly pour the liquid. Comments:	☐	☐	☐	
8. Replace the cap on the bottle. Comments:	☐	☐	☐	
9. Write the date and time the container was opened on the label of the bottle or a piece of tape. Comments:	☐	☐	☐	

Checklist for Procedure 149 Applying and Removing Sterile Gloves

Name _____ Date _____

School _____

Instructor _____

Course _____

Procedure 149 Applying and Removing Sterile Gloves	Able to Perform	Able to Perform with Assistance	Unable to Perform	Initials and Date
1. Wash your hands. *Comments:*	☐	☐	☐	
2. Check glove package for sterility. *Comments:*	☐	☐	☐	
3. Use your thumbs to peel back the upper edges of the outer package. *Comments:*	☐	☐	☐	
4. Remove the inner package containing the gloves. *Comments:*	☐	☐	☐	
5. Place the inner package on the inside of the outer package. *Comments:*	☐	☐	☐	
6. Open the inner package. *Comments:*	☐	☐	☐	
7. Use your left hand to pick up the cuff of the right-hand glove. *Comments:*	☐	☐	☐	
8. Insert your right hand into the glove. *Comments:*	☐	☐	☐	
9. Insert the gloved fingers of your right hand under the cuff of the left glove. *Comments:*	☐	☐	☐	
10. Slide your fingers into the left glove. *Comments:*	☐	☐	☐	

continued on the following page

continued from the previous page

Procedure 149	Able to Perform	Able to Perform with Assistance	Unable to Perform	Initials and Date
11. Adjust each glove for comfort. *Comments:*	☐	☐	☐	
12. Insert your right hand under the cuff of the left glove. *Comments:*	☐	☐	☐	
13. Push the cuff of the left glove over your wrist using your gloved right hand. *Comments:*	☐	☐	☐	
14. Insert your left hand under the cuff of the right glove. *Comments:*	☐	☐	☐	
15. Push the cuff of the right glove over your wrist using your gloved left hand. *Comments:*	☐	☐	☐	
16. To remove your gloves, grasp the outside of the glove on your nondominant hand at the cuff. *Comments:*	☐	☐	☐	
17. Pull the glove off, keeping the inside of the glove facing outward. *Comments:*	☐	☐	☐	
18. Place this glove into the palm of the gloved hand. *Comments:*	☐	☐	☐	
19. Put the fingers of the ungloved hand inside the cuff of the gloved hand. *Comments:*	☐	☐	☐	
20. Pull the glove off inside out. *Comments:*	☐	☐	☐	
21. Discard the gloves according to policy. *Comments:*	☐	☐	☐	
22. Wash your hands. *Comments:*	☐	☐	☐	

Checklist for Procedure 150 Using Transfer Forceps

Name _____ Date _____

School _____

Instructor _____

Course _____

Procedure 150 Using Transfer Forceps	Able to Perform	Able to Perform with Assistance	Unable to Perform	Initials and Date
1. Wash your hands. *Comments:*	☐	☐	☐	
2. Open the package of sterile supplies. *Comments:*	☐	☐	☐	
3. Grasp the needed item with the tips of the forceps. *Comments:*	☐	☐	☐	
4. Pick up the item. *Comments:*	☐	☐	☐	
5. Move the item to the sterile field. *Comments:*	☐	☐	☐	
6. Lay the tips of the forceps within the sterile field. *Comments:*	☐	☐	☐	
7. Keep the handles outside the sterile field if they are to be reused. *Comments:*	☐	☐	☐	

Checklist for Procedure 151   Head-Tilt, Chin-Lift Maneuver

Name _____ Date _____

School _____

Instructor _____

Course _____

Procedure 151 **Head-Tilt, Chin-Lift Maneuver**	Able to Perform	Able to Perform with Assistance	Unable to Perform	Initials and Date
1. Place one hand on the forehead. *Comments:*	☐	☐	☐	
2. Place the fingers of the opposite hand below the center of the jawbone, directly under the chin. *Comments:*	☐	☐	☐	
3. Tilt the head back gently. *Comments:*	☐	☐	☐	
4. Lift the jaw forward with your fingertips. *Comments:*	☐	☐	☐	
5. Keep the patient's mouth open and, if necessary, manually maintain this position. *Comments:*	☐	☐	☐	
6. As soon as other professionals have assumed care, wash your hands. *Comments:*	☐	☐	☐	

Checklist for Procedure 152   Jaw-Thrust Maneuver

Name _____ Date _____

School _____

Instructor _____

Course _____

Procedure 152 Jaw-Thrust Maneuver	Able to Perform	Able to Perform with Assistance	Unable to Perform	Initials and Date
1. Move the patient into a supine position. *Comments:*	☐	☐	☐	
2. Pull the head of the bed away from the wall. *Comments:*	☐	☐	☐	
3. Position yourself above the patient's head. *Comments:*	☐	☐	☐	
4. Place your elbows on the mattress. *Comments:*	☐	☐	☐	
5. Use your forearms to stabilize the sides of the head. *Comments:*	☐	☐	☐	
6. Place one hand on each side of the lower jaw. *Comments:*	☐	☐	☐	
7. Push the lower jaw forward with the tips of your index fingers. *Comments:*	☐	☐	☐	
8. Keep the patient's mouth open and, if necessary, manually maintain this position. *Comments:*	☐	☐	☐	
9. As soon as other professionals have assumed care, wash your hands. *Comments:*	☐	☐	☐	

Checklist for Procedure 153 Mask-to-Mouth Ventilation

Name _____ Date _____

School _____

Instructor _____

Course _____

Procedure 153 Mask-to-Mouth Ventilation	Able to Perform	Able to Perform with Assistance	Unable to Perform	Initials and Date
1. Pull the head of the bed away from the wall. *Comments:*	☐	☐	☐	
2. Apply disposable gloves. *Comments:*	☐	☐	☐	
3. Open the patient's airway. *Comments:*	☐	☐	☐	
4. Position yourself at the patient's head. *Comments:*	☐	☐	☐	
5. Position the mask on the patient's face. *Comments:*	☐	☐	☐	
6. Seal the mask to the patient's face and hold the airway in the open position. *Comments:*	☐	☐	☐	
7. Take a deep breath. *Comments:*	☐	☐	☐	
8. Seal your mouth over the ventilation port and exhale into the mask. *Comments:*	☐	☐	☐	
9. Check for rise of the patient's chest during ventilation. *Comments:*	☐	☐	☐	
10. Remove your mouth from the mask and allow the patient to exhale passively. *Comments:*	☐	☐	☐	
11. Breathe into the mask once every 4 to 5 seconds. *Comments:*	☐	☐	☐	

Checklist for Procedure 154   Adult CPR, One Rescuer

Name _____ Date _____

School _____

Instructor _____

Course _____

Procedure 154 Adult CPR, One Rescuer	Able to Perform	Able to Perform with Assistance	Unable to Perform	Initials and Date
1. Gently shake the person and ask, "Are you okay?" *Comments:*	☐	☐	☐	
2. Call for help. *Comments:*	☐	☐	☐	
3. Turn the victim on his back as a unit. *Comments:*	☐	☐	☐	
4. Open the airway and place your ear near the patient's mouth. *Comments:*	☐	☐	☐	
5. Observe the victim's chest for movement. *Comments:*	☐	☐	☐	
6. Look, listen, and feel for 3 to 5 seconds. *Comments:*	☐	☐	☐	
7. If no signs of breathing are found, seal the victim's nose with your thumb and forefinger and seal the victim's mouth using your mouth or barrier device. *Comments:*	☐	☐	☐	
8. Ventilate 2 times, taking 2 seconds for each ventilation. *Comments:*	☐	☐	☐	
9. Allow the chest to deflate between ventilations. *Comments:*	☐	☐	☐	
10. Check for the presence of a heartbeat for 5 to 10 seconds. *Comments:*	☐	☐	☐	

continued on the following page

continued from the previous page

Procedure 154	Able to Perform	Able to Perform with Assistance	Unable to Perform	Initials and Date
11. If there is a pulse but no respirations, continue with ventilations. *Comments:*	☐	☐	☐	
12. If there is no pulse, begin chest compressions. *Comments:*	☐	☐	☐	
13. Do four cycles of 15 compressions to 2 ventilations per cycle. *Comments:*	☐	☐	☐	
14. At the end of four cycles, feel for the carotid pulse for 5 seconds. *Comments:*	☐	☐	☐	
15. If no pulse, ventilate 2 times. *Comments:*	☐	☐	☐	
16. Continue the cycle of 15 compressions to 2 ventilations. *Comments:*	☐	☐	☐	
17. Feel for the carotid pulse every few minutes. *Comments:*	☐	☐	☐	
18. If victim resumes breathing but is unconscious, place in recovery position on his side. *Comments:*	☐	☐	☐	
19. If the heart is beating but there is no breathing, continue ventilations at a rate of 1 every 5 seconds or 12 times per minute. *Comments:*	☐	☐	☐	
20. If there is no heartbeat and no breathing, continue with chest compressions and ventilations at the ratio of 15 compressions to 2 ventilations. *Comments:*	☐	☐	☐	

Checklist for Procedure 155   Adult CPR, Two Rescuer

Name _____ Date _____

School _____

Instructor _____

Course _____

Procedure 155 Adult CPR, Two Rescuer	Able to Perform	Able to Perform with Assistance	Unable to Perform	Initials and Date
1. With CPR in progress, a second rescuer comes in after a cycle of 15 compressions and 2 breaths is completed. *Comments:*	☐	☐	☐	
2. One rescuer should move to the victim's head, open the airway, say "Stop CPR," and check for return of pulse. *Comments:*	☐	☐	☐	
3. Other rescuer finds the correct hand position. *Comments:*	☐	☐	☐	
4. If pulse is absent, say "No pulse." *Comments:*	☐	☐	☐	
5. Ventilator gives 2 breaths and compressor begins chest compressions. *Comments:*	☐	☐	☐	
6. Count compressions as one and two and three and four and five. *Comments:*	☐	☐	☐	
7. At the end of the 15th compression, the compressor should pause for the ventilator to give 2 breaths. *Comments:*	☐	☐	☐	
8. Continue the cycle with periodic pulse checks. *Comments:*	☐	☐	☐	
9. If both rescuers arrive at the same time, one rescuer should call EMS while the other begins one-rescuer CPR. *Comments:*	☐	☐	☐	

continued on the following page

continued from the previous page

Procedure 155	Able to Perform	Able to Perform with Assistance	Unable to Perform	Initials and Date
10. One rescuer checks for respirations while the other finds the correct location for chest compressions. *Comments:*	☐	☐	☐	
11. Ventilator should monitor the pulse during the cycle. *Comments:*	☐	☐	☐	
12. Compressor gives 15 compressions at the rate of 100 a minute. *Comments:*	☐	☐	☐	
13. Ventilator gives 2 ventilations. *Comments:*	☐	☐	☐	
14. Continue the cycle until victim regains consciousness or you are exhausted and unable to continue. *Comments:*	☐	☐	☐	
15. Stop chest compressions for 5 seconds at the end of the first minute and every few minutes thereafter to check for pulse and respirations. *Comments:*	☐	☐	☐	
16. Change positions without interrupting the 15:2 sequence. *Comments:*	☐	☐	☐	
17. Rescuer performing compressions directs the switch. *Comments:*	☐	☐	☐	

Checklist for Procedure 156   Positioning the Patient in the Recovery Position

Name _____ Date _____

School _____

Instructor _____

Course _____

Procedure 156 Positioning the Patient in the Recovery Position	Able to Perform	Able to Perform with Assistance	Unable to Perform	Initials and Date
1. Kneel beside the patient and straighten his legs. *Comments:*	☐	☐	☐	
2. Place the arm nearest you above the patient's head with the palm up and elbow bent slightly. *Comments:*	☐	☐	☐	
3. Position the patient's opposite arm across his chest. *Comments:*	☐	☐	☐	
4. Place your lower hand on the patient's thigh on the far side of the body. *Comments:*	☐	☐	☐	
5. Pull the thigh up slightly, closer to the center of the patient's body. *Comments:*	☐	☐	☐	
6. Roll the patient onto his side facing you. *Comments:*	☐	☐	☐	
7. Move the patient's upper hand close to the cheek. *Comments:*	☐	☐	☐	
8. Adjust the upper body so the hip and knee are at right angles. *Comments:*	☐	☐	☐	
9. Tilt the patient's head back slightly. *Comments:*	☐	☐	☐	
10. Place the patient's upper hand palm down under the cheek to maintain the head position. *Comments:*	☐	☐	☐	
11. Continue to monitor the patient. *Comments:*	☐	☐	☐	

Checklist for Procedure 157   Heimlich Maneuver–Abdominal Thrusts

Name _____ Date _____

School _____

Instructor _____

Course _____

Procedure 157 **Heimlich Maneuver–Abdominal Thrusts**	Able to Perform	Able to Perform with Assistance	Unable to Perform	Initials and Date
1. Ask the person if she is choking. *Comments:*	☐	☐	☐	
2. If she starts to cough, wait. *Comments:*	☐	☐	☐	
3. If the person cannot speak, cough, or breathe, stand behind the victim and wrap your arms around the victim's waist. *Comments:*	☐	☐	☐	
4. Clench your fist, keeping the thumb straight. *Comments:*	☐	☐	☐	
5. Place your fist against the abdomen above the navel and below the tip of the xiphoid process. *Comments:*	☐	☐	☐	
6. Grasp your clenched fist with your opposite hand. *Comments:*	☐	☐	☐	
7. Thrust forcefully inward and upward. *Comments:*	☐	☐	☐	
8. Keep thrusting until the obstruction is expelled or the victim becomes unconscious. *Comments:*	☐	☐	☐	

Checklist for Procedure 158   Assisting the Adult Who Has an Obstructed Airway and Becomes Unconscious

Name _____ Date _____

School _____

Instructor _____

Course _____

Procedure 158 Assisting the Adult Who Has an Obstructed Airway and Becomes Unconscious	Able to Perform	Able to Perform with Assistance	Unable to Perform	Initials and Date
1. Activate the EMS system. Comments:	☐	☐	☐	
2. Apply disposable gloves. Comments:	☐	☐	☐	
3. Turn the victim on his back. Comments:	☐	☐	☐	
4. Grasp victim's tongue and jaw between your thumb and fingers. Comments:	☐	☐	☐	
5. Pull upward to open the mouth and draw the jaw forward (tongue-jaw lift). Comments:	☐	☐	☐	
6. Insert the index finger of your opposite hand down along the inside of one cheek, toward the base of the tongue. Comments:	☐	☐	☐	
7. If you can see the object, use a hooking motion to loosen and remove the object. Comments:	☐	☐	☐	
8. If the object is brought into the mouth, remove it. Comments:	☐	☐	☐	
9. If the victim is not breathing, give one slow breath. Comments:	☐	☐	☐	
10. If the air does not go in, reposition the head and try again. Comments:	☐	☐	☐	

continued on the following page

continued from the previous page

Procedure 158	Able to Perform	Able to Perform with Assistance	Unable to Perform	Initials and Date
11. If the air still does not go in, straddle the victim and give 5 abdominal thrusts. *Comments:*	☐	☐	☐	
12. If the obstruction is not removed, continue to repeat the procedure until the obstruction is removed or more advanced health care professionals arrive. *Comments:*	☐	☐	☐	
13. If the obstruction is removed, keep the airway open and check for breathing. *Comments:*	☐	☐	☐	
14. If not breathing, provide rescue breaths at a rate of one every 5 seconds. *Comments:*	☐	☐	☐	

Checklist for Procedure 159 CPR for Infants

Name _____ Date _____

School _____

Instructor _____

Course _____

Procedure 159 CPR for Infants	Able to Perform	Able to Perform with Assistance	Unable to Perform	Initials and Date
1. Determine unresponsiveness by tapping the shoulder. *Comments:*	☐	☐	☐	
2. Call out for help. *Comments:*	☐	☐	☐	
3. Support the infant's head and shoulders and place the infant on his back on a firm surface. *Comments:*	☐	☐	☐	
4. Open the airway using the head-tilt, chin-lift maneuver. *Comments:*	☐	☐	☐	
5. While maintaining an open airway, position your head over the infant's chest and look, listen, and feel for breathing. If the infant is breathing and there are no signs of trauma, place the infant in the recovery position. *Comments:*	☐	☐	☐	
6. If the infant is not breathing, maintain an open airway and give two slow, gentle breaths with your mouth completely covering the infant's nose and mouth. *Comments:*	☐	☐	☐	
7. Assess circulation by checking for the brachial pulse. *Comments:*	☐	☐	☐	
8. If there is no pulse, begin chest compressions by positioning your index and middle finger one finger-width below the nipple line in the center of the sternum. Compress the sternum $\frac{1}{2}$ to 1 inch at a rate of 100 per minute. *Comments:*	☐	☐	☐	
9. Give 5 compressions and one breath. Repeat until 20 cycles are complete. *Comments:*	☐	☐	☐	

continued on the following page

continued from the previous page

Procedure 159	Able to Perform	Able to Perform with Assistance	Unable to Perform	Initials and Date
10. Reassess the brachial pulse. *Comments:*	☐	☐	☐	
11. Activate the EMS system if this has not already been done. *Comments:*	☐	☐	☐	
12. If there is no pulse, continue compressions and rescue breaths. *Comments:*	☐	☐	☐	
13. Reassess for pulse after each 20 cycles or when the infant's condition appears to change. If a pulse is present, reassess for breathing. If the infant is not breathing, continue rescue breathing. If there is no pulse, continue CPR. *Comments:*	☐	☐	☐	

Checklist for Procedure 160　Obstructed Airway: Conscious Infant

Name _____ Date _____

School _____

Instructor _____

Course _____

Procedure 160 Obstructed Airway: Conscious Infant	Able to Perform	Able to Perform with Assistance	Unable to Perform	Initials and Date
1. Determine if there is an airway obstruction by observing breathing difficulties, weak or absent cry, or ineffective cough. *Comments:*	☐	☐	☐	
2. While supporting the infant's head and neck with one hand, position the infant on one arm, face down with head lower than the trunk. *Comments:*	☐	☐	☐	
3. Deliver up to 5 back blows. *Comments:*	☐	☐	☐	
4. Turn the infant face up and deliver up to 5 chest thrusts at a rate of 1 per second. *Comments:*	☐	☐	☐	
5. Repeat back blows and chest thrusts until foreign body is expelled or the infant becomes unconscious. *Comments:*	☐	☐	☐	
6. If the infant becomes unconscious, call for help and activate EMS. *Comments:*	☐	☐	☐	
7. Place the infant on his back. *Comments:*	☐	☐	☐	
8. Perform a tongue-jaw lift. Remove any visual foreign body, but do not sweep blindly. *Comments:*	☐	☐	☐	
9. Open the airway with the head-tilt, chin-lift. *Comments:*	☐	☐	☐	

continued on the following page

continued from the previous page

Procedure 160	Able to Perform	Able to Perform with Assistance	Unable to Perform	Initials and Date
10. Attempt rescue breaths. *Comments:*	☐	☐	☐	
11. If breaths do not go in, reposition the head and try again. *Comments:*	☐	☐	☐	
12. If breaths still will not go in, deliver up to 5 back blows. *Comments:*	☐	☐	☐	
13. Deliver up to 5 chest thrusts. *Comments:*	☐	☐	☐	
14. Perform a tongue-jaw lift and remove the foreign body if you can see it. *Comments:*	☐	☐	☐	
15. While maintaining an open airway, try again to give rescue breaths. *Comments:*	☐	☐	☐	
16. Repeat until successful: open airway, attempt breaths, back blows, chest thrusts, tongue-jaw lift, attempt breaths. *Comments:*	☐	☐	☐	
17. If alone, activate EMS after one minute. *Comments:*	☐	☐	☐	
18. Once the obstruction is cleared, check for breathing. *Comments:*	☐	☐	☐	
19. If not breathing, give 2 rescue breaths. *Comments:*	☐	☐	☐	
20. If no pulse, begin CPR with a ratio of 5 compressions and 1 breath. *Comments:*	☐	☐	☐	
21. If there is a pulse but the infant is not breathing, continue by giving 1 rescue breath every 3 seconds and monitor pulse. *Comments:*	☐	☐	☐	

Checklist for Procedure 161   Obstructed Airway: Unconscious Infant

Name _____ Date _____

School _____

Instructor _____

Course _____

Procedure 161 Obstructed Airway: Unconscious Infant	Able to Perform	Able to Perform with Assistance	Unable to Perform	Initials and Date
1. Determine unresponsiveness. *Comments:*	☐	☐	☐	
2. Call for help. *Comments:*	☐	☐	☐	
3. Support the head and neck and turn the infant on her back on a hard, firm surface. *Comments:*	☐	☐	☐	
4. Open the airway using the head-tilt, chin-lift method. *Comments:*	☐	☐	☐	
5. Determine lack of breathing by maintaining an open airway and looking, listening, and feeling for breathing. *Comments:*	☐	☐	☐	
6. Attempt to give rescue breaths by placing your mouth over the infant's nose and mouth. *Comments:*	☐	☐	☐	
7. Reposition the head, check your mouth seal, and attempt rescue breaths again. *Comments:*	☐	☐	☐	
8. Activate the EMS system. *Comments:*	☐	☐	☐	
9. Deliver up to 5 back blows. *Comments:*	☐	☐	☐	
10. Deliver up to 5 chest thrusts. *Comments:*	☐	☐	☐	

continued on the following page

continued from the previous page

Procedure 161	Able to Perform	Able to Perform with Assistance	Unable to Perform	Initials and Date
11. Do a tongue-jaw lift and remove the foreign body if visible. *Comments:*	☐	☐	☐	
12. Attempt rescue breaths again. *Comments:*	☐	☐	☐	
13. Repeat back blows, chest thrusts, jaw lift, and rescue breaths until successful. *Comments:*	☐	☐	☐	
14. Activate the EMS system after one minute of effort. *Comments:*	☐	☐	☐	
15. Check for pulse and respirations when the obstruction is removed. *Comments:*	☐	☐	☐	
16. If the infant is breathing, place in recovery position. Maintain open airway and monitor pulse and breathing. If there is no breathing, give 1 rescue breath every 3 seconds and monitor the pulse. *Comments:*	☐	☐	☐	
17. If there is no pulse, give 2 rescue breaths and start cycles of compressions and breaths. If there is a pulse, open the airway and check for breathing. *Comments:*	☐	☐	☐	

Checklist for Procedure 162   CPR for Children, One Rescuer

Name _____ Date _____

School _____

Instructor _____

Course _____

Procedure 162 **CPR for Children, One Rescuer**	Able to Perform	Able to Perform with Assistance	Unable to Perform	Initials and Date
1. Establish unresponsiveness by tapping the shoulder and calling the child's name. *Comments:*	☐	☐	☐	
2. If another person is available, ask that person to activate the EMS system. If no one else is present, perform CPR for 1 minute, and then activate EMS. *Comments:*	☐	☐	☐	
3. Open the airway using the head-tilt, chin-lift method. *Comments:*	☐	☐	☐	
4. Check for breathing by looking, listening, and feeling for breath. If the child is breathing, place the child in the recovery position. *Comments:*	☐	☐	☐	
5. If the child is not breathing, give 2 slow breaths. Allow for passive exhalation. *Comments:*	☐	☐	☐	
6. Check a carotid pulse. If pulse is present but patient is not breathing, give 1 rescue breath every 3 seconds. *Comments:*	☐	☐	☐	
7. If there is no pulse, locate the landmark by using an imaginary line between the nipples. Place the heel of one hand on the middle of the sternum one finger-width below this line. *Comments:*	☐	☐	☐	
8. Give 5 chest compressions at a rate of 100 per minute and a depth of 1 to $1\frac{1}{2}$ inches. *Comments:*	☐	☐	☐	

continued on the following page

continued from the previous page

Procedure 162	Able to Perform	Able to Perform with Assistance	Unable to Perform	Initials and Date
9. Open the airway and give 1 breath. *Comments:*	☐	☐	☐	
10. Repeat the cycle of 5 compressions to 1 breath 20 times. *Comments:*	☐	☐	☐	
11. Reassess the patient after 20 cycles or one minute. *Comments:*	☐	☐	☐	

Checklist for Procedure 163   Child with Foreign Body Airway Obstruction

Name _____ Date _____

School _____

Instructor _____

Course _____

Procedure 163 Child with Foreign Body Airway Obstruction	Able to Perform	Able to Perform with Assistance	Unable to Perform	Initials and Date
Conscious Child				
1. Ask child if she is choking. *Comments:*	☐	☐	☐	
2. If yes, position yourself behind the child. *Comments:*	☐	☐	☐	
3. Wrap your hands around the child and place one fist between the xiphoid process and the navel. *Comments:*	☐	☐	☐	
4. Roll the thumb end of the fist into the patient's abdomen and provide quick upward thrusts with the intent of forcing remaining air out of lungs. *Comments:*	☐	☐	☐	
5. Repeat until foreign body is removed or victim becomes unconscious. *Comments:*	☐	☐	☐	
If the Child Becomes Unconscious...				
6. Ask someone to activate EMS. *Comments:*	☐	☐	☐	
7. Perform a tongue-jaw lift and remove any foreign body you see. *Comments:*	☐	☐	☐	
8. Open the airway and attempt rescue breathing. *Comments:*	☐	☐	☐	
9. If the breath will not go in, reposition the head and try again. *Comments:*	☐	☐	☐	

continued on the following page

continued from the previous page

Procedure 163	Able to Perform	Able to Perform with Assistance	Unable to Perform	Initials and Date
10. Straddle the child's thighs and give 5 upward abdominal thrusts. *Comments:*	☐	☐	☐	
11. Repeat steps 7–10 until successful. *Comments:*	☐	☐	☐	
12. If obstruction not relieved after 1 minute, activate the EMS system. *Comments:*	☐	☐	☐	